Gender, power and change in health institutions of the European Union

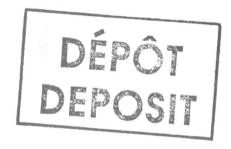

DÉPÔT
DEPOSIT

Paola Vinay — Prospecta, Ancona

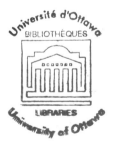

Employment & social affairs

Equal opportunities and family policy

European Commission
Directorate-General for Employment, Industrial Relations
and Social Affairs
Unit V/D.5

Manuscript completed in April 1997

This report was financed by and prepared for the use of the European Commission, Directorate-General for Employment, Industrial Relations and Social Affairs. It does not necessarily represent the Commission's official position.

It is a synthesis of:
Paola Vinay — Prospecta, April 1997, *Women in decision-making in the health institutions of the European Union* — European Commission V/5806/97-EN.

Chapter 1 was written by Massimo Paci; chapters 2 to 5 by Paola Vinay.

Cover picture: 'Training little medics' — 'Pictures by Chinese children', Foreign Languages Press, Peking, 1976.

A great deal of additional information on the European Union is available on the Internet.
It can be accessed through the Europa server (http://europa.eu.int).

Cataloguing data can be found at the end of this publication.

Luxembourg: Office for Official Publications of the European Communities, 1997

ISBN 92-828-1362-2

Printed in Belgium

Table of contents

Preface

The aim of the research presented here was to analyse the access of women to senior decision-making positions in the health institutions of the 15 EU Member States and at European Union level. Only the public health sector was covered, including "semi-public" institutions such as mutual health associations or sickness funds, but leaving apart the private sector, which anyhow is in a minority in all EU countries. More precisely, the access of women to the following institutions was studied:
- main political bodies (Ministry of Health; Parliamentary Health Committees; Regional Political Authorities);
- central administrative institutions (Directorates General of the Ministry of Health; top positions within public health insurances or funds);
- main national medical unions or associations;
- main consultative and bargaining bodies in the health sector;
- top management of the five largest hospitals of each country.

This study presupposes a basic understanding of the functioning of the national health systems of EU Member States. The first task of the study, therefore, was to describe the 15 countries' health systems and build up a "map" of the main health institutions in each one of them.

The main focus of the study, though, is on the obstacles to adequate representation of women and on their role in health decision-making. This objective was pursued in three steps. First of all, with the crucial contribution of the national experts of the European Network "Women in Decision-Making", we collected the available data on male-female participation in high-level positions. We were thus able to make a list of about one thousand women in top-level positions in the 15 EU health systems. Secondly, we mailed a questionnaire to these women (and to an equal number of men, in the same positions), in order to collect information on the factors which prevent a higher participation by women in decisional power and on their role in health.

Thirdly, we made a "qualitative study" in Sweden, France and Italy, by doing a limited number of "open" interviews with women occupying top positions in the health sector. These three countries were chosen because they represent fairly well the three main types of health systems prevailing in the European Union today: Sweden represents the "universal" model prevailing among the Northern European countries of the Union, while France is representative of the "occupational" model shared by most of the Central European countries, and Italy represents the "mixed" type of health system (in transition from the "occupational" type towards the "universal" one) which characterizes the Southern European Member States.

Finally, in the general conclusions we discuss some policy proposals.

Chapter 1

HEALTH INSTITUTIONS IN THE EU MEMBER STATES

1.1 Models of health systems

Every EU country operates facilities designed to protect or to optimize public health in respect of such matters as sanitation, water supplies and food hygiene. All of them, furthermore, possess a quantity of statutory medical facilities in the form of public hospitals along with local public or community health medical personnel. This being said, there are nevertheless significant differences between the various health systems of the EU countries.

One explanation is to be found in the ways in which the different European societies have attempted (or refrained from) regulation of patient-health services interaction. The first important stage in health policy development, from Bismarck onwards, was for particular categories of the population to be singled out for favoured treatment, through the introduction of the first schemes of social insurance. (The employed in particular came to attract such attention). The next step, taken mainly after World War II with varying degrees of abruptness among European countries, consisted of moving from categorial (or "occupational") to population-wide or "universal" policy coverage (Flora-Heidenheimer, 1981).

Two main "models of coverage" can be identified: the "occupational" (or "corporatist") model and the "universal" (or "statutory") one. In the universal (or statutory) model the main subject of public coverage is the citizen: all citizens are covered in the same way irrespective of their work or family position, while the financial support comes from taxation on general revenues. Where this model is historically rooted (like in Sweden or in the United Kingdom for instance), it has engendered national systems of compulsory health insurance or national health services, directly managed by the State. In the occupational (or corporatist) model the subject of coverage is not the citizen, but the worker paying contributions from earned income to "sickness funds" (or similar "third party" insurers), according to his/her employment category, while the non-active population has eventually acquired the right to coverage either as retired workers or as dependent members of the breadwinner's family. (Germany and France, for instance, have historically developed this model).

Moreover, those states in which the universal model of coverage prevails (Sweden, Denmark, United Kingdom, Ireland, and - to a lesser extent - Finland), are also those in which the principal source of financing is taxation on general revenues. On the contrary, contributions paid to sickness funds constitute the most common source of financing in those states in which the occupational model of coverage prevails (Austria, Germany, France, Belgium, Netherlands and Luxembourg).

3

Nevertheless, there are some exceptions to this trend. In fact, the Southern European countries (Greece, Italy, Portugal and - to a lesser extent - Spain), though they have - according to their laws - a universal model of coverage, still rely upon a high amount of contributions to finance their systems. Moreover, in Southern European countries, the national health service "contracts out" to private centres (the Spanish *conciertos*, the Italian *centri convenzionati*) the provision of a vast array of services: from diagnostic tests to minor or medium surgery (Ferrera, *1995*). For these countries, thus, we may identify a "mixed" model of coverage: this is formally universal or "statutory", but, in fact, it draws an important proportion of its financing from the contributions paid by occupational groups and "sub-contracts" many public care services to private providers.

Another significant institutional feature of the health system is the range of devolution of power to sub-national authorities. In Sweden, on one side of the spectrum, government of health is highly decentralized both functionally and geographically: the county councils, for instance, levy their own health taxes. In France, despite important recent efforts to decentralize, the health administration remains unitary and centralized: local political authorities have only minor responsibilities in health care matters. On the contrary, in Germany and in Italy the sub-national authorities have their own separate health administration.

The description of the health systems of the 15 EU countries, provided in the previous pages, can be summarized in a scheme of synthesis, with reference to the model of coverage and the range of devolution of decisional power to sub-national authorities (see fig. 1).

Fig. 1 - **Distribution of the health systems of the EU Member States according to the model of coverage and the range of devolution of power to sub-national authorities**

Model of coverage	Range of devolution	
	high	*low*
"Universal":	Denmark, Finland, Ireland, Sweden	United Kingdom
"Occupational":	Austria, Belgium, Germany	France, Luxembourg, Netherlands
"Mixed":	Italy, Portugal*, Spain*	Greece

* Partial devolution .

4

1.2 Social and political actors

Many social and political "actors" play a role on the national health scene. Central political authorities, of course, (i.e. the Ministry of Health, and the Parliamentary Health Committees) are crucial. But also high-level administrative authorities (for instance, the heads of the main departments of the Ministry), and (where existing) the autonomous regional (or county) political authorities play an important role in health politics and policies. The same can be said for many "bargaining" organizations such as the national medical associations and the unions representing health employees and employers. The sickness funds are still important in some countries, although they are restricted increasingly to an administrative role. Hospitals too, particularly public "regional" ones, are important centres of power at a local level. Finally, the constellation of «consultative bodies» (set up by governments as "advisory" committees or as representatives of vested interests) also have an influence upon policy-making in health. The growth of these bodies has been fostered by the need to manage the conflicting interests of the State, employers and workers.

A synthetic description of the institutional framework and governing bodies of the health system is given in fig. 2.

Fig. 2 - **Institutional framework and governing bodies of the health system.**

	Policy making	Public administration	Semi-public administration and financing	Consultation and bargaining
National level	Central political authorities (*Ministry of Health, Parliament Health Committees*)	Central health administration (*Directors Gener.*)	Health insurance agencies and sickness funds (*Execut. boards*)	- Consultative bodies (*members*) - Medical associations and unions (*Executive boards*)
Regional level	Local political authorities (*same as at the national level*)	- Main Public hospitals (*board of trustees*)		

While the Minister of Health is chosen by the Prime Minister, the members of the Parliamentary Health Committees are selected by the parliamentary groups and, in the last analysis, by the deputies belonging to the various political parties in the Parliament (The same can be said, of course, for the regional political authorities). We may call this the "political channel" to high-level decision-making in health.

As far as the "consultative bodies" are concerned, their members may be politicians, civil servants, representatives of interest organizations or "experts". They are set up, usually, by the Ministry itself. They may be chosen either as individuals, holders of specific expertise in health matters, or as individuals incorporated in organizations designed to further important interests in health.

5

We may call this the "corporatist channel" to high level decision-making in health[1].

The main Directors of the various administrative departments (or "divisions") of the Ministry of Health are usually selected through promotion from the inner grades of the administrative structure, and this is, of course, the "bureaucratic channel" to high level positions in health. (In some countries, though, the Directors general of the Ministry of Health are appointed by the Minister, who may choose them from outside the administrative structure).

Within the "semi-public" administrative bodies, such as sickness funds (or other similar compulsory insurance agencies) the selection of personnel to high level positions (chair, deputy-chair and members of the executive boards) may follow either the "bureaucratic channel" or the "corporatist" one: in fact, the top management of the sickness funds may be chosen from the high grades of the administration of the funds themselves or among the representatives of specific vested interests (such as the insurers and insured people, i.e. the employers' and the workers' organizations).

Finally, selection to decision-making positions in public hospitals may follow either the "political" or the "corporatist" or the "bureaucratic" channel, and the chair of the executive board may be a physician serving as medical director, a civil servant or a business manager.

In this chapter, we have analysed the models of coverage and financing and the degree of devolution of power among the 15 health systems of the EU Member States[2]. We have identified also the main health institutions and the "channels" to the decision-making positions inside them. It will be interesting to verify - at the end of our study - how the representation of women in the decision making-process in the health sector is influenced by these institutional features.

---

[1] Gaining access to decision-making positions through the "corporatist channel" seems more difficult for women. Out of a total of 171 "advisory bodies" of all Dutch ministries, surveyed in 1987, the average percentage of female members was as low as 10,5%, that is: "... considerably lower than the participation of women in most other parts of the political system in the Netherlands" (Oldersma, 1992, p. 4).

[2] For a brief description of the health system of each Member State on the basis of which this synthesis was made, see M. Paci, in Vinay-Prospecta, 1997, chapter 2.

Chapter 2

WOMEN IN HEALTH EMPLOYMENT AND DECISION-MAKING

2.1 Women's employment in the health sector

Noticeable differences exist among the Member States of the European Union in the access of women to the formal labour market and particularly to non-traditional "feminine" occupations. In spite of the rapid change underway, there is still considerable disparity in equal opportunities for women among the Southern and the Northern countries of the Union. However - as the research work of the European Network "Women in Decision-Making" shows - similarities persist among all the Member States which inhibit equal opportunities for women in the access to top positions and to decisional power.

Employment in health has been growing significantly in the last twenty years in all Member States. Between 1970 and 1990 employment in this sector tripled or nearly tripled in Italy and Greece, doubled or nearly doubled in Germany, Finland, Sweden and Portugal and increased considerably also in the United Kingdom, Ireland and Denmark. This sharp increase has favoured the employment of women everywhere. In 1981-82 women already constituted the majority of health workers in all the 15 EU Member States. The problem is whether this general employment growth also improved the access of women to top level and managerial positions.

Today women have attained levels of education higher than those of men and are represented in the whole range of the health professions. In all EU countries, women account for more than 60%, often two-thirds, of total health employment. Our study, though, concerns the top positions, i.e. the centre of power and decision-making in health, and in this field in all EU countries their participation is still far from adequate.

Traditionally physicians have an important decisional power in health policies and administration. From this point of view we may consider the rate of women physicians as a first rough indicator of the participation of women in medium-high level positions. In the last decades the number of women physicians has increased in many countries. In Finland, for instance, 65% of the 1992 new PhDs in medicine were women, and in France the percentage of women among students of medicine rose from 44 to 50% between 1982-83 and 1993-94. In spite of this increase in the number of women physicians, up to now the ratio of women physicians to all physicians is still lower than 50% in all EU countries. Disparity among the Member States is strong: the lowest ratios are in Belgium and Italy were women are not even reach 25% of all physicians. The highest ratios are found in Finland (42.4%), Portugal (40%) and Sweden (34%); in all the other countries these ratios are between 26% and

30%. The range of disparity among the Member States is as high as twenty percentage points.

The gender disparity in employment may be even sharper if we consider in detail the professional groups involved in the health sector. If the top positions are analysed in more detail, women are found towards the bottom, particularly in the professional groups that do have decisional power: often their numbers as head physicians and administrative top managers are very low. For instance, within the 208 local health units of the Italian national health service, only 2.9% of the directorates general, 4.5% of the management directorates and 8.4 of the health care directorates are entrusted to women. The same happens within hospitals, where only 3.6% of directors general, 4% of management directors and 11.8% of health care directors are women. In Austria, according to 1994 data of the national medical order, women were 46% of training physicians, 34% of all general practitioners and 26% of consultants. Similar data are reported for Germany: in 1992-93 women were 45% of university students of medicine, 35% of all practising physicians, but only 5% of chief physicians.

As far as the different professional groups are concerned the share of women is higher among biologists, psychologists, physio-therapists and everywhere they form the majority of nurses and other non-medical health professionals. For instance, in Spain, although women make up over 60% of all the personnel employed in the national health service, INSALUD, the proportion of women doctors is 28%, while the proportion of women in other health care professions is as high as 98%. In France, women are 28% of practising general practitioners, but they are about 75% of psychologists-psychoanalysts, rehabilitation and diet staff, 85% of chief nurses and almost 100% of midwives and infant care staff.

In the United Kingdom, women constitute 78% of the personnel of the national health service and 89% of the non-medical staff. Between 1984 and 1994 the percentage of women physicians rose from 23 to 30%, but only from 13 to 18% among consultants. Also in the United Kingdom, the percentage of women varies according to the different medical specializations: in 1994, for instance, women were only 7% of surgeons (i.e. the same percentage as in 1984), while they were about 50% of paediatricians. Similarly, in Ireland, women are 39% of psychiatrists, but only 3% of surgeons. In Sweden, finally, as in the other countries, women predominate in psychology (74%), physiotherapy (88%) and nursing, but they are only 25% of senior physicians.

These data show that in health, as in other economic branches, women - in spite of the changes undergone in the last twenty years - seem to find a "glass ceiling" above them even when they reach the top positions.

2.2 Women in decision-making positions

The rate of women in high-level decisional positions is still far from being equal to that of men in most EU countries. The information gathered by the

Network members in 1996 made it possible to fill out several "country tables" with the number of men and women in the highest decision-making positions in the 15 EU countries. An analysis of these data shows that in the majority of them, women are strongly under-represented. There are wide differences, though, particularly among the type of health institution and "cultural area" of Europe (North, Centre or South) considered.

a) *Political institutions*
Women are relatively better represented in political bodies than in administrative institutions, though there are noticeable differences among the EU Member States. We may recall, first of all, a good result: as many as nine of the 15 Ministers of Health of the Union are women (in 1996). Taking into account, on the whole, the Ministry of Health, the "under-secretaries" of the Ministry and the members of the Parliamentary Health Committees, the percentage of women is higher than 50% in five of the 15 EU countries (Sweden, Finland, Denmark, Netherlands and Germany), 45% in Ireland, and between 32 and 40% in 4 other countries (Belgium, Spain, United Kingdom and Austria), while it is lower than 25% in Luxembourg, France, Italy, Portugal and Greece.

Table 1 - **Central political authorities (Government and Parliament): distribution by sex of top positions in the European Union and in its 15 Member States, 1996**

Countries	GOVERNMENT				PARLIAMENT				COMMITTEES %W	TOTAL %W
	Minister		*UnderSecr*		*Chair*		*Members*			
	M	F	M	F	M	F	M	F		
Denmark	-	1	1	-	-	1	13	15	54	**53**
Finland	-	1	2	-	1	-	11	15	58	**55**
Ireland	1	-	1	-	1	1	19	17	47	**45**
Sweden	-	1	5	14	1	-	8	8	50	**64**
U.K.	1	-	3	1	-	1	7	5	42	**35**
Austria	-	1	-	3	1	-	25	13	34	**40**
Belgium	-	1	1	-	1	1	22	10	31	**32**
France	1	-	1	-	2	-	169	23	12	**12**
Germany	1	-	2	1	1	1	21	27	56	**54**
Luxemb.	1	-	8	4	1	-	10	1	10	**21**
Netherl.	-	1	2	2	-	2	18	19	51	**52**
Greece	1	-	2	-	1	-	49	3	6	**5**
Italy	-	1	10	4	1	1	55	16	23	**24**
Portugal	-	1	1	-	1	-	18	3	14	**17**
Spain	-	1	5	2	1	1	47	21	31	**32**
E. U.					1	-	25	20	44	

Source: European Network "Women in Decision-Making", our data processing.

9

If we refer to the twenty-three Parliamentary Committees which have authority on health matters, we may see (in table 1) that women chair nine of them. Moreover, in five EU countries (Finland, Denmark, Sweden, Netherlands and Germany), women are 50% or more of the members of these Committees. The percentage is slightly higher than 40% in the United Kingdom and in the European Parliament, while it drops in all the other countries, reaching particularly low percentages in Portugal (14%), France (12% before the 1997 elections), Luxembourg (10%) and Greece (6%). We shall recall, for this purpose, that - as was shown by the survey on Women in Decision-Making in Political Institutions - the representation of women in the Parliamentary Health Committees is higher than in the other parliamentary committees of the EU Member States. We must remember too that the European elections of 1994 brought a steady increase in the representation of women within the European Parliament (from 19.5 to 25.6%) and, hence, within the parliamentary committee which has authority on health matters (from 26.8 to 44.4%). This increase was the result of the awareness raising campaign promoted by the European Network under the agreements of the Athens Conference. In some European countries, however, the representation of women within the Parliament has remained very low or decreased (as in Italy in the 1996 elections).

b) *Central health administration*

To compare women's representation in the administrative institutions of the health sector in the 15 EU Member States is more difficult. There is a wide cross-country variation in the organization of the state health administrations. Women are less well represented in administrative decision-making on health than in policy making. The general directorates and vice-directorates of state administration in the health sector are usually entrusted to men. Women are more present at the level of the administrative "divisions", but they are still under-represented (see table 2). More precisely, not a single woman is to be found at the level of the "directorates general" (i.e. at the highest level of the state administration) in one third of the EU countries (Finland, Austria, Belgium, Netherlands and Italy). Taking into account also the "vice-directorates" and the directorates of the divisions, the percentage of women exceeds 35% in six countries (Sweden, Finland, France, Luxembourg, Italy and Portugal). This percentage is, however, lower than 22% in Austria, Belgium, Germany and the Netherlands. (The representation of women is rather scant, moreover, within the directorates of the Council and the Committee of the European Parliament dealing with health matters).

Women are very under-represented also at the top levels of the sickness funds and mutual associations in all the EU countries where such "semi-public" institutions exist and play an important role. In this case, the highest percentage of women in decision-making positions is in Belgium (22%), while in the other countries it is always under 15% and as low as 5% in Germany.

c) *Hospitals and local administrative authorities*

Also within hospitals and the main local health authorities, men predominate in decision-making positions. The percentage of women among the top managers of the five largest hospitals of each EU country is almost everywhere lower than 40%.

Table 2 - **Central Health Administration: distribution by sex of the directorates general, sub-directorates, directorates of divisions of the Ministry of Health and National Health Insurance and of Sickness Funds, 1996**

MINISTRY OF HEALTH AND N. H. INSURANCE

	Direct.Gen.		Sub-Direct.		Dir.Division		Total		
Countries	M	F	M	F	M	F	M	F	%W
Denmark	4	3	2	-	59	10	65	13	17
Finland	7	-	6	4	32	24	45	28	38
Ireland	18	5	36	14			54	19	26
Sweden	6	5	5	9			11	14	56
Austria	3	-	3	-	3	-	9	-	0
Belgium	6	-	12	1	125	23	143	24	14
France	4	2	-	1	3	1	7	4	36
Germany	8	1	12	-	83	19	103	20	16
Luxemb.	5	8	8	1			13	9	41
Netherl.	9	-	11	2	25	10	45	12	21
Greece	8	3					8	3	27
Italy	7	-	2	5	23	15	32	20	38
Portugal	10	2	11	10			21	12	36
Spain	8	2	25	13			33	15	31
E.U.	2	1	3	-	12	2	17	3	15

SICKNESS FUNDS & MUTUAL ASSOCIATIONS

	Chair		Deputy-chair		Total Members		%W
Countries	M	F	M	F	M	F	
Belgium	2	-	1	-	35	10	22
France	3	-	6	1	96	14	13
Germany	12	-	13	-	158	8	5
Luxemb.	9	-	7	2	74	7	9
Netherlands	1	-	2	-	7	-	0
Greece	9	1	10	-	147	28	16

Source: European Network "Women in Decision-Making", our data processing.

d) *The advisory or consultative and bargaining bodies*
In the top positions of this kind of institution, women are often a very small minority. Only Sweden, Denmark and Ireland are exceptions, with 40% of women or more (see table 3). As far as the national medical unions or associations are concerned, men outnumber women by far (once more with the exception of Sweden). As a matter of fact, in order to acquire representation women physicians, have established their own international professional association.

Table 3 - National Advisory, Consultative bodies and National Medical Associations: distribution by sex of members, 1996

Countries	CONSULTATIVE and ADVISORY BODIES Chair M	F	Members M	F	% W	MEDICAL ASSOCIATIONS and BARGAINING BODIES Chair M	F	Members M	F
Denmark	5	1	66	44	40	4	-	9	-
Finland	1	-	5	3	38	3	2	9	6
Ireland			40	31	44			82	14
Sweden	2	3	25	22	47	1	1	15	16
U.K.			1.520	710	32				
Austria	1	-	22	-	0	2	-	5	2
Belgium	3	-	9	2	18	2	-	19	-
France	5	2	249	31	11	3	1	162	19
Germany	1	-	6	1	14	3	1	33	16
Luxemb.	5	-	74	4	5	5	-	25	2
Netherlands	3	1	180	15	8				
Greece	1	-	45	8	15	4	1	83	11
Italy	2	-	80	5	6	4	1	203	17
Spain	3	-	27	5	16	3	-		81
								28	
E.U.	4	-	12	3	20				

Source: European Network "Women in Decision-Making", our data processing.

2.3 Women in decision-making by major European regions

As shown in Chapter 1, European health systems can be differentiated into three major models according to their institutional features: the Northern European countries (Denmark, Ireland, Finland, Sweden and United Kingdom) are characterized by a "universal" system; the Central European countries (Austria, Belgium, France, Germany, Luxembourg, and the Netherlands), have a variety of health insurance schemes, along "occupational" (and sometimes denominational) lines administered by "semi-public" bodies, such as the sickness funds or mutual associations; finally, the Southern European countries (Greece, Italy, Portugal and Spain) are characterized by a "mixed" model of health protection. The data we gathered show that the participation of women in decision-making is higher among the five "universal" systems of state protection of the Northern European countries. In this case, the women's participation rate is higher than 45% within political bodies, 35% within advisory or consultative bodies, and than 25% within administrative institutions in four of the five countries.

Women representation decreases, however, among the six "semi-public" and "occupational" systems of the Central European countries. In this case, women exceed 45% within the political bodies only in two of the six countries; they never exceed 30% within the advisory or consultative bodies, while they exceed 25% within the administrative institutions only in two of the six countries. Particularly low, in all these countries, is the representation of women in the top positions of the sickness funds, mutual associations and national medical associations.

The representation of women, finally, is lowest among the four "mixed" systems of the Southern European countries, with the exception of public administrative institutions, where this same representation exceeds 25% in all four countries of this group.

In conclusion, women's participation in decision-making in health is related to the model of the health system prevailing in each country. It is encouraged by the public "universal" systems of Northern European countries. In the "mixed" systems of the Southern European countries, though women are generally under-represented in decision-making, the recent transition towards the "universal" model of health protection seems to result in an increase of women's representation within the public administrative institutions of the health sector. Finally, it is worth noting that, among Central European countries, even where women's representation is relatively high in the political bodies, it is often low within the advisory or consultative bodies and within administrative "semi-public" institutions.

Chapter 3

THE SURVEY: THE ROLE OF WOMEN IN HEALTH

Up to this point, analysis has shown that in most European countries women are still greatly under-represented in decision-making bodies, even though they make up a large part of health employment and in spite of the fact that the number of women at higher levels has substantially increased. Why is it that so few women are present in decision-making processes in this sector, and what are the main obstacles for a balanced presence of men and women? These questions have been answered through a wide survey, with questionnaires mailed to both women and men holding high decisional positions in the health institutions of the 15 EU countries identified in the first part of the study. This has been done with the crucial help of the European Network "Women in Decision-Making", which supplied us with the names and addresses. 398 persons answered the questionnaire: 220 women and 178 men.

Physicians - particularly chief physicians - are very much represented in our sample, and this is particularly true for men: 40% of men (and 26% of women) are physicians. Moreover, 32% of men are chief-physicians (but this is true for only 18% of women). On the contrary, nurses and other non-medical health professions are represented mainly by women. (As a matter of fact, 17% of the women in the sample are nurses or belong to non-medical health professions, while this happens to only 6% of men). We find relatively more women than men also in professions such as "clerks", "teachers" and "self-employed", particularly in political bodies. It is worth noting, moreover, that the women of our sample are much younger than the men. For both sexes, the age bracket most represented is the 45-54 years one. But, while, the share of those younger than 45 years are 39% of the female sample, this happens only to 18% of the men.

3.1 The role of selection and promotion criteria

The first important data of the survey is that only 4% of the 220 women who answered the questionnaire (and 12% of men) felt that there were no obstacles to the presence of women in decision-making in health policy. The others, instead, referred to more than one obstacle.

Selection criteria for access to decision-making bodies and to important tasks within the body can be an obstacle to women. It is so, for example, for an unspecifically objective criterion like "aptitudes for management", mentioned by over a third of women and men. We should, at this point, ask what criteria establish whether one has an "aptitude for management", if for example, importance is attributed to the ability to give orders which are then blindly followed, or if instead, factors such as the ability to cooperate, listen to other people's suggestions, make shared decisions, are looked for. (In fact, our study shows that there are differences between men and women in the style of leadership).

Another criterion which is frequently mentioned by the respondents of both sexes, is previous experience (in the present body or in other public or private ones); this criterion can penalize women, not only for a presumed lesser experience given the average lower age, but rather for the fact of having made their career in areas considered "less important or sectorial". (This is an obstacle mentioned by 14% of men and by 31% of women).

More interviewed women than men also declared that belonging to a political party, trade union or an organized group is often a selection criterion. Obviously belonging to a political party mainly refers to political bodies. However the criterion of belonging to a party, trade union or movement, is identified - above all by women - also referred to management bodies in which it should not be taken into account. This criterion is frequently found also in advisory or consultative and bargaining bodies: in both cases the percentage of women is at least double that of men. (In particular, while half the number of men are members of a political party, this is true of only 6% of their female colleagues). It is also important that a large number of women - higher than the number of men - refers to "political acquaintances" or "other influential people" as an important factor for access to decision-making roles both in central health and hospital management bodies, and in consultation and advisory ones. It is therefore not surprising that many women feel that "not knowing influential people" is to be included among the main obstacles to female presence in decision-making.

Among the main criteria for access and attribution of tasks in health decision-making bodies (above all in local and national management), the one mentioned most frequently is the level of education: more than two thirds of the respondents referred to this. In fact, nearly all respondents have a university degree, there are however differences as to the type of degree: while over half of the men have a degree in medicine, this is true for slightly more than a third of women. Compared to men, double the number of women have a degree in classical studies (12.4% compared to 5.8%) and nearly five times the number a degree in psychology (5.9% compared to 1.4%) or a university diploma in nursing, social work or physiotherapy (15.4% compared to 2.9%).

This would suggest intervention in women's choice of education. But one should also ask if there are no unjustified rigidities in this field. If, for example, a degree in medicine is really preferable in health decision-making and in hospital management or if experience in social and caring work is not just as important. (In fact, in some Member States those who are responsible for nursing services are on the management advisory board of hospitals). Often reality seems to be similar to the description of a German respondent :

> *"The physicians are mostly men and the nurses women. When it is necessary to take a decision the male physicians think they are "superior" to the female nurses".*

If selection and promotion criteria mentioned up to now are obstacles for an equal representation of women, it is not surprising that nearly a third of the respondents

(32%) feels, that to reach a more equal division of decisional power, it is necessary to change these criteria and 17% of them believe that a quota in favour of women should be introduced. Other measures which are often mentioned refer to updating and special training programmes (23%), institutional programmes for equal opportunities (30%) and improvement of information channels on career opportunities (17%).

3.2 The role of family care

Other important obstacles depend largely on the difficulty of combining both professional and family life. In fact 68% of women and 65% of men who answered the questionnaire identified "personal ties and family responsibility", as among the most important obstacles to women's access to decision-making roles, ties which often result in - according to 37% of women and 35% of men - insufficient motivation for a career.

Where this is concerned it must be pointed out that actually one third of the women interviewed is "single" or "divorced", (nearly three times the number of men). Besides, nearly a third of them has no children and another 20% has only one child (the percentages for men are considerably lower in both cases: 13 and 16%). This demonstrates that without adequate social services, and a more equal division of family duties between sexes and in the presence of rigid work organization, only women with fewer family ties find less obstacles in their access to decision-making roles.

It therefore follows, that measures deemed suitable to deal with this kind of problem include courses aimed at increasing women's self-esteem (according to 30% of female respondents and 21% males), at improving social services - as underlined by 28% women and 27% men - but, above all, at intervention on working time schedules (such as flexible working hours, work-sharing, possibility to organize work by oneself): as much as 60% of women and men referred to this type of intervention. One Belgian respondent, for example, felt it was necessary to have longer parental leaves. One Swedish woman summarizes the problem in the following way:

> "Measures are required to lighten the work load of women who have a job and family responsibilities, such as greater equality between husband and wife at home and a general reduction of work hours".

3.3 Discriminating practices and appreciation of competence

At this point, a very important data must be underlined, also because it is stressed with the same frequency by both sexes. Over a third of interviewed women and men, mentions that relevant obstacles to the presence of women in decision-making are the diffusion of prejudices and discriminating practices against women. Moreover, the questionnaires show that these practices are present even against women who have reached important decision-making roles.

Certainly most of the women - and men - who answered the questionnaire do not, in any way, feel discriminated against or that their competence is not appreciated enough. These are people, however, who have already reached the highest levels and therefore should not have any particular reasons not to be satisfied. But also at these levels we register signs of discomfort and persisting symptoms of discrimination. In fact, a no mean number (15%) of female respondents experienced some discrimination since being part of that body. This, actually, occurred most frequently in hospitals (23%). Here are the testimonies of an Italian and a Danish women:

"In various public examinations I experienced quite evident unfairness against which I was "ungrateful" enough to rebel".

"Some visitors from other hospitals asked themselves if a woman was capable of being senior consultant; sometimes male colleagues make ironical remarks".

Most respondents - women and men - find no difference between duties given to men and those given to women. However, many women (24%) - independently of their age group - feel that in their place of work there is a difference, in the sense that men have more qualified positions and selection criterion at all levels favour them, while women are taken into consideration only for specific tasks. Here, for example, are the replies of an Italian, French and Finnish woman:

"The greatest differences are access exclusion to managerial functions or to representation of executive bodies and exclusion from top managerial positions".

"Men have more support in obtaining high positions".
"Women often have positions as experts or consultants, men are heads of units or departments".

In fact, 42% of women experience obstacles in carrying out their role within the body. This is true for 37% of men, although the kind of obstacle faced is considerably different: it is more often a political or bureaucratic one for men and, instead, more often a lack of resources, information, support from their superiors and of credibility attributed to their gender for women. Of course, these obstacles are perceived more by the younger respondents, but the greatest difference between men and women (over 10 percentage points) can be found in the older age brackets. This negative perception, in the case of women, is most frequently found in hospitals: 53% of women in hospital management committees (compared to 37% of men) feel partially prevented from carrying out their decisional role. These are the answers of two German respondents and a woman from Luxembourg:

"I'm a woman and a nurse whose work is not fully accepted by the dominant medical staff".

"There is bad organization and bad information about decision-making processes".

"There is a lack of moral and material support from the superiors".

Many complain that the authority their work carries is not recognized and that their competence is not sufficiently valued. In fact, over 27% of women (10 percentage points more than men) feels that their competence is not properly appreciated. This occurs with the same frequency for all age groups, while in the male group it is mostly the younger men who feel this. Lastly 31% of women - young or old and independently from whatever body they belong to - feel that their opinion is not taken into sufficient consideration. Also a significant number of men (24%)

complain about this, though once again, in their case this usually concerns the younger ones and those working in political bodies. Again, the greatest difference between men and women regarding this problem can be found in the hospital environment: 35% of women with decision-making roles in hospitals feel that their opinion is not taken into sufficient consideration with a difference of 21 percentage points compared to men. Two answers, one from a German respondent and one from an Italian, illustrate this point:

"The fact that I'm a female nurse and not a male doctor means that many male heads of department don't take me seriously at first and I have to waste a lot of time convincing them".

"To get some results, you have to make continually greater efforts to assert yourself, which is often exhausting".

Given these premises it is not surprising that most women who answered the questionnaire - over 58%, nearly 10 percentage points more than men - were relatively unsatisfied regarding the effective decision-making power they had due to: the scarce power of the body itself, the reduced possibilities of people acting within that body, the excessive bureaucratic or hierarchic conditioning, and also to the presence of prejudices which create inequality. (It must be noted that while in the case of men yet again it's the young ones who are disappointed, in the case of women this is true of both young and old). It therefore follows that a smaller number of women than men hope to get, in the near future, a position of greater responsibility (and a greater number of men has already reached the top offices in the body) in spite of the fact that for more women than men, the main reasons which drove them to be part of the body in the first place, were the possibility of making a career and of having a position of greater prestige and responsibility.

We will conclude this paragraph with some sentences which explain the delusion of some women respondents:

"The position of political "advisor" of the Minister is often vague, I would like to have more specific responsibilities" (Sweden).

"It is very difficult for women to succeed in being part of commissions which make political decisions" (Germany).

"I'm disappointed because it is a body which does not affect the decision-making process, but only the final phase. Discussions on this are always conditioned by decisions already made by the different political parties" (Italy).

"Progress is very fragmentary, interests of the medical and health operator corporations are far too involved; there is no consistency in the choice of quality opportunities for the citizens" (Italy).

3.4 Similarities and differences among major European regions

From the analysis, it seems quite clear that, still today, selection criteria in leading decision-making health bodies favour men. Even those women who are able to break through the "glass ceiling" and reach the summit, find that they have to face difficult situations and make personal sacrifices much more than their male colleagues. We will now look at the similarities and differences among three geographical-cultural areas which are the North, Centre and South of Europe.

These areas - as previously shown - are characterized by different systems of health protection, both institutionally and regarding the participation of women in decision-making.

Our survey showed that - in spite of the geographical-cultural area they come from - women often have similar characteristics and opinions which are quite different from men's. For example, everywhere at least double the percentage of women than men believes that to have a balanced presence of women in decision-making processes in health, it is necessary to change the selection and promotion criteria. Everywhere, they have more often a university diploma rather than a degree or post-graduate qualification. They also, more often than men, believe that an unobjective criterion such as "management aptitude" is one of the main criterion with which posts are given; everywhere twice as many women, than men, believe that women are at a greater disadvantage because they have made their career in sectors (or disciplinary areas) which are traditionally deemed less important. Also women in the North, Centre and South, compared to their male colleagues, have more difficulties even within the decision-making body in which they work, as they believe that there are systematic gender differences in the distribution of tasks and responsibilities, that men are given more prestigious positions and that women's opinion is not given sufficient consideration.

However, in spite of the numerous similarities, there are also very significant differences. Compared to women in the Centre and South, women (and men) in North of Europe more often mention experience in the health sector, and education qualification as access criterion and for task attribution in the body they belong to. It should be noted that the North registered the highest number of women and men with a university diploma, which means that in this area even they have access to decision-making roles.

Compared to women in North and Centre of Europe, many more women in the South (53% compared respectively to 30% and 33%) identify, as one of the main obstacles to access of women to decision-making roles, the presence of prejudices and discriminating behaviour against them. Declarations of having been discriminated against are more numerous (21%) and a higher proportion of women believe that they don't have career possibilities.

Another important difference is given by the fact that, compared to the ones in the North, a much higher number of women in Centre and South of Europe identifies family responsibilities as one of the main obstacles for women in decision-making. Besides, women in the Centre and South of Europe who have reached top decision-making roles, much more often than their colleagues from the North, are "single" or separated and without children or with only one child: 47% of the female respondents in the South doesn't live as a couple, double the number of those in the North; 39% of them has no children and 29% has only one child, while two thirds of the women in the North have at least two children. It should be noted that, contrary to women, very few men in the South (only 9%) do not live as a couple, while this percentage rises a little in the North (16%) where the difference between men and women is greatly reduced.

From this data analysis we can draw the conclusions that not having a family seems to be, in the Central and Southern European countries (much more often than in the North), a factor which favours women's careers at a higher level. It is therefore understandable that these women believe, more often than in the North, that improving social services is one of the main factors to help women's participation in decision-making. (This is true for 47% of women in the South, compared to 19% in the North).

3.5 Reasons for the participation of women in health policy choices

Let us see now, using the sample survey, why is an adequate participation of women in health decision-making important, and whether they contribute in a new and valuable way.

According to 41% of men who answered our questionnaire, "competence" seems to be the only important factor in the decisional process of health policies. This percentage falls to 22% for women, the majority of whom (54%) believe that gender is just as important as competence. Another 24% of them (like 22% of men) considers the presence of women as "important" or "fundamental".

As to the reasons for these answers, it must be said that the respondent didn't refer only to a principle of equity, but also (above all for women) to the fact that women have a different way of confronting health problems, of viewing reality and have a wider experience of caring problems. Here is the opinion of some women who answered the questionnaire:

> *"Competence is important because health is an extremely complex sector; the female presence is important because women in the "government of public things" are seen to be competent, sensitive, attentive to other people's needs, willing to listen and able to mediate" (Italy).*

> *"Without life experience (and mine is the experience of a woman's life) it is not possible to work well" (Germany).*

> *"Competence is always important and sometimes women have a kind of experience and competence that men don't have" (Sweden).*

Besides, 62% of men and 68% of women believe that in bodies where health decisions are taken, it is "necessary" or "fundamental" to have specific competence in female problems. These, for example, are some of the reasons given:

> *"Specific competence in women's problems is necessary because certain needs of the female psychology can be better expressed" (Spain).*

> *"For a better understanding of specific problems" (Holland).*

> *"Competence in women's problems can help to give a more global and adequate approach" (Italy).*

"It is important because women have other priorities and recognize the risk of medicalizing women and the relative invisibility of women's health" (Denmark).

3.6 The role of women's experience of life

Some of the above replies refer to the different way women related themselves to health problems. This fact becomes even clearer from the answers to a specific question. In fact, 70% of the female respondents believe that women have different views on health policies, above all due to their different experience of life and because they look after the family.

"I believe that women have different experiences and priorities: I think that women are more interested in prevention and men more in treatment" (Sweden).

"As women have a different experience of life and different health problems from men, their opinion can contribute to a diverse and more universal approach" (Germany).

The opinions reported here are widespread among women, both in the North, Centre and South of the Union. Apart from their geographical-cultural area or the kind of national health system, women have similar opinions regarding their role in health, which often differ from men's. Thus, for example, women who believe that only competence is important are much fewer than men everywhere, while in all countries the majority feel that specific competence in female problems is important. It isn't only for a democratic principle that women believe that the presence of their gender is important in bodies which decide national health policies.

On the other hand, due to the very fact that they make up the majority of health operators and users of health services, women have developed a considerable experience about the functioning (and dysfunctions) of the health system. Based on daily experience, they have developed an approach to health problems which better meets the needs of the population.

It is also common knowledge, that most of the common health problems in the family are faced without any kind of professional help: "self-help" and "self-care" are, in fact, very diffused in all European countries. Women have always been given the responsibility of family planning, of looking after the family, children, elderly, and disabled, thus substituting the socio-health services. Also because of the responsibility which has historically and culturally been laid on their shoulders regarding eating habits, personal and environmental hygiene, health promotion of both themselves and their family, women have acquired the kind of knowledge which makes them particularly sensitive to prevention.

It is, therefore, logical that in answer to the question "What are the most important health policy measures", a significantly higher percentage of women than men (55% compared to 42%) refers to integration of social and health services, to services for the elderly and to improving the quality of services. Similarly a higher number of women refers to prevention, health education and participation (60% compared to 48%). (A greater number of men, instead, refers to waste control and rationalization of public expenditure).

21

3.7 Changes in men's attitude

We should ask ourselves, at this point, whether a larger presence of women in decision-making would bring about a change in the general direction of health policies. In fact, in those bodies where actions have been taken promoting the presence of women to tasks of responsibility, these initiatives not only increased the presence of women in the body, but also led to changes in the style of argumentation, in decisional methods and in health policy management, producing changes in men's behaviour towards women.

In those countries where the presence of women in high decision-making positions is more consistent, men have a much more positive attitude towards women regarding the importance of women in health. In Northern European countries - where there are more initiatives promoting the presence of women to tasks of responsibility - the percentage of men who believe that only competence is important in the health sector, drops to 29%, while it is over 50% in the Centre and 42% in the South. Also, compared to the Centre and South, the majority of men in the North feel that specific competence of women's problems is necessary (69%) and also believe that women have a different way of dealing with health problems (47%). The experience of sharing work with women, seems to bring about changes in men's attitudes towards them. It is interesting to note that men in the North seem much less worried than their colleagues in the Centre and South about controlling health expenditures.

It may be useful, where this point is concerned, to give the replies of some men from Sweden, which is the most advanced European country regarding equal representation of sexes in decision-making in the public health sector :

> "It is important to look at health problems from two different angles".

> "Women's way of thinking and experience are different from men's and it is important that both be represented".

> "Women are important in all caring activities. The point of view of both sexes is necessary".

To conclude, our survey shows that a more balanced presence of women in the bodies with decisional power for health is important not only for a question of equity in representation, but also, and above all, because woman bring new values, new ideas and a new style and method in decisional process. Besides, in those countries where, for some time now, women have played an important role in decision-making processes, men's attitude has changed in their favour. Obviously, the latter have had a chance to appreciate the importance of women's innovative contribution in the field of health policy.

We shall conclude this chapter with a sentence from one of our interviews:

> "Women are much more willing to confront themselves, they are less governed by the logic of belonging (either to a party or to a corporation), much "freer" to understand and decide on the basis of general interest" (Italy)

Chapter 4

WOMEN, POWER AND INNOVATION: A QUALITATIVE STUDY IN FRANCE, ITALY AND SWEDEN

In this chapter we shall look at the results of the third part of the research, which is a qualitative study of three European countries representative of the three geographical-cultural areas. The three chosen countries are: Sweden for the Northern countries, characterized by a "universal" model of welfare system, France for Central Europe which has an "occupational" health insurance system, and Italy for the Southern countries where the universal health protection system is incomplete or "mixed". As already shown in the previous chapters, these geographical-cultural areas, and especially the countries chosen, present different levels of female representation in decision-making; but strong similarities in the women's attitude regarding their role in public health. The 16 in-depth interviews which we shall analyse here elaborate the main themes which emerged in the sample survey, and that is: the importance of women's role in this sector; their innovative contribution, and useful suggestions to foster female representation.
Before analysing the replies to these important subjects, we shall briefly compare the three chosen countries on the basis of some indicators of health efficiency.

4.1 Some indicators of health efficiency

Infant mortality and perinatal rates are usually considered as valid indicators of health efficiency. In all Western countries these rates have drastically fallen in this century as a result of perinatal prevention, improved hygienic conditions and medical assistance at birth and during the first days of life. However, conditions and services still vary considerably, even among European countries. According to the OCSE data of 1990-91, Sweden - with 0.61 per cent of live births - presents the lowest infant mortality rate in Europe; this rate increases for France with 0.73% and reaches 0.83% for Italy - this last percentage is lower only to the one for Belgium, Greece, Luxembourg and Portugal.

Regarding maternity safety, a recent French publication of the Haut Comité de la Santé Publique (1995) reported, that in the '70s France made considerable progress where perinatal mortality was concerned, but since 1985 has marked time, with the result that now it is in 13th place among the OCSE countries. Moreover, a third of the death of mothers (14 per 100.000), could be avoided. According to the Committee the reasons for these high rates can be attributed, to insufficient or bad quality assistance at the moment of birth, to delay in diagnosis and in resolving complications both in the mother and child.

Another indicator of medical efficiency is the percentage of ceasarian births out of the total number of births. Sweden has the lowest rate out of the three countries considered and among the lowest in Europe (following only Ireland and Great Britain) and this rate is decreasing considerably in the last ten years. Italy, on the contrary, has the highest rate in Europe and it continues to rise. The rate for

France is in an intermediate position compared to the European countries, but it is rising there too. It must be noted, that the percentage of ceasarian births is much lower in all Northern European countries, in which the health protection system is universal and the presence of women in decision-making is higher. In the other European countries, instead, these percentages are not only higher but, above all in the South, they tend to rise.

The indicators of medical efficiency mentioned here concern health problems which specifically involve women. It is, therefore, not wrong to relate them to the greater or lesser presence of women in decision-making processes in health in the various countries. Another important indicator, on this matter, is prevention of breast cancer and cancer of the womb. According to the Haut Comité de la Santé Publique, between 1950 and 1990, while mortality from stomach cancer - which mainly affects men - greatly decreased in France, in the same period mortality from breast cancer increased significantly (in 1991 ten thousand women in France died from this disease). Prevention campaigns, especially mammography for women in menopause has made it possible to cut the mortality by 30%, but this examination has only recently begun to be performed over the whole French territory. Even mortality prevention from cancer of the womb is badly used in France: only a minority of women, especially those most at risk, are controlled, and this is a clear symptom of, at least, insufficient information.

To conclude, these data demonstrate both some differences among the three countries in medical efficiency and that where there is a greater presence of women with decisional roles in health, also conditions are more favourable for safety in maternity and of the new-born and there is more health protection towards both woman and child.

4.2 Biographical profiles of women in decision-making

a) The Italians
For the in-depth interviews a Southern Italian city was chosen where there is a group of women with decisional roles in the health sector who, for some time now, have been paying particular attention to specific female problems. Here below is a brief personal profile of the five women we interviewed.

1 - Elsa is a psychologist who has reached the top level in her profession and is director of a mental health operating unit. Married, she began to have disagreements with her husband when her child was born and she separated. "At the beginning of my career - she says - the idea of equality helped me ("I'm like you, if you can then I can"), then differences emerged during maternity, my being a woman. Besides, the director had to choose between me and a man and he chose the man although I was more competent. This helped me to understand the situation better and at this point I upheld the women's banner. When I became senior consultant I invented work inside the Service which didn't exist before: a "Health for Women" sector, which is not foreseen, which legally doesn't exist, so I'm an inexistent director of an inexistent structure, an invention, and I can practise the power of fact which is not legal power. My experience began within Democratic Psychiatry, but we had to admit that in this reform the men would

forget specific women's problems: when the psychiatric hospitals opened, the only ward which didn't open was the one for mentally ill women, because the problem of sexuality had to be resolved". Together with a group of women Elsa took the reponsibility of opening the doors of the women's ward and looking after the health of the female patients, delegating only the specific role to the physician.

2 - Grazia co-ordinates the maternity-infant operating unit of her city. Graduated in medicine at only 23, specialised in cardiology, she began a university career which she then abandoned because of family problems: married, she has 5 children. "My university career was equal, but problems started when I began to have a family, because of the hours: I needed to have regular schedules, but when you work on experiments you come home when you have finished. So with my second child I had to abandon university. I went to work in the Office of Hygiene which had daytime hours, so I had a little space, very limited, in which to be a doctor and I had to be grateful for just that. My family greatly limited my capacities, I had to accept a role which wasn't really what I wanted, but neither did I want to give up my children and husband. My husband had space for his career, he never had problems with time, he didn't have to curb his career with hours". Grazia has also other reponsibilities: she teaches at a school for health operators; she is part of the regional study group which gives advice to operators working in the maternity-infant sector. As far as she is concerned, she has managed to train continuously and this is what has helped her.

3 - Anna, senior consultant in psychiatry, is responsible for a unit of mental health. She is married and has two children. For some years she worked with female patients, participating, with a group of women in creating a Women's Service within the Mental Health Service. Since 1993 she is a senior consultant: "This position was accepted well, above all by the operators (there are many women). The directors had more difficulty accepting it: in meetings there were only men with typically male language, and embarassment which was mostly theirs". Anna has had various kinds of training: psychotherapy, epidemiological research, management course. She is now president of a management association which she herself created, to promote initiatives for the organization and promotion of quality services. She was helped in her career by "great will-power, stubbornness, desire for challenge.. which has been very tiring, perhaps too much so, and has brought about a situation of stress".

4 - Paola, biologist, research director in an international centre of research on molecular surgery. She is also a member of EMBO (European Molecular Biology Organization) and in Italy is responsible for a special Cancer Research Association project on tumoral angiogenesis. She works in medical research: angiogenesis, cancer, embrional development. Some years ago she isolated a gene involved in blood capillary growth. Among other things she is a CEE referee in evaluation of research projects in her field. She spent three long study and work periods in the United States. When she returned to Italy she immediately got a place as a senior consultant. She is divorced and has a daughter whom she took to the States with her : "My daughter was 5 years old - she says - only a woman can do so many things: be a mother, organize her family and at the same time organize a laboratory, carry out research; I'd like to see if a man can do as much... I divorced

because my husband was not willing to go halves in looking after his daughter and the house; I had to look after my daughter completely and also after him, so I said "please go away". I then realized that I had more free time to dedicate to my daughter, my work and my friends".

5 - Ivana, councillor for social services, before the Conference of Rome she formed a work group on themes regarding women and health which gave rise to work proposals and food for thought. This group collaborates with the Women's Centre of her city, a centre which receives and connects initiatives of women's associations.

b) The French

1 - Michéle, member of the national council of an association of general practitioners in France, representative of the Comité de Liaison des Femmes Médecins (committee of the union of women physicians). She has a surgery of general medicine and is also very active in the association. Besides, in her area she is involved in permanent medical training, organizes seminars both locally and nationally, participates in evening meetings among local general practitioners and specialists. Married with a small child, she believes that being a woman did not hinder her career but helped her to become more determined. About the association of general practitioners she says: "This union was born 10 years ago when we women entered the labour market... we shaped it to our image; we chose the right moment, one in which women's voices were being listened to. Before this, I was part of a group of women physicians who had got together to face practical problems such as, keeping a surgery going even when you were having a child, we then all joined the union where, compared to other medical associations, women play an important role. For ten years I worked alone as a general practitioner, but since my daughter was born five years ago, I joined other women general practitioners and mothers, and opened a surgery with them, which we could run much better together".

2 - Catherine, runs one of the 52 hospitals in Paris; she mentions that in the area of Paris many hospital directors are women - more than elsewhere - because the role of director in this case is more that of an executor, as these hospitals are subordinated to the "Hopitaux de Paris" institution which is the real decision-making place. Catherine's training and professional experience was deeply affected by family problems, as she says "a divorce was necessary to build a professional career". She interrupted her doctorate in law because she married a diplomat and went to live abroad: for 12 years could not hallow her own career. After her divorce, while working she began to study again passing the exam of the National School of Health to become hospital director. This exam - she says - is very difficult for women: "There are always many women for the written part and many of them pass because it is anonymous, but selection occurs in the oral part where certainly more men pass". It was very hard for her to work and study, as Catherine has two children, one by her first husband and one by her current companion. Even he has not helped her much, in fact when she had to move to another city for her courses, the youngest child should have stayed with the father, but he complained that this was incompatible with his work and so she had to take the little one with her.

3 - Danielle, is also a hospital director and has a similar professional-family experience to Catherine. She studied German and Russian, then human sciences, but had to interrupt her doctorate to follow, with a child, her husband; she had to move yet again to follow her husband, but also wanted to work and continue her studies. She then moved once more to follow a course and this time her husband had to follow her. But, when she presented for political elections, her husband was unable to endure her life rhythm and they divorced. Also Danielle, after the divorce, went to the National School of Health and won a place as hospital director. About this she says: "My class was the first one where as many women as men passed, but there was a violent reaction to this by the profession who said that the profession would lose its value if it was womanized, so in the following years a smaller number of women passed this exam. I'll give you an example: there are 91 psychiatric hospitals in France, but only 7 women directors, even though many are vice-directors".

4 - Thérèse, is chair of a national association of gerontology, retired head of the Direction National de la Santé, she received a Legion d'Honneur medal. Divorced with grown children, she states that in France statistics demonstrate a growing number of women who want divorce, because they have less need of the material security given by marriage. She underlines the importance of her mother on her training: "As my mother was a very independent woman, I wasn't brought up with the idea of necessarily having to get married, but with the idea of having a profession and being independent: I was educated to have aims in my life, just like a boy".

5 - Jacqueline, additional general secretary of one of the most important national federation of mutual associations, is employed in a sickness fund, now detached for union activity in the national federation. She only finished primary school: "I trained in the field - she says - I usually say that I did my university studies in the union". I have always worked in a very serious way and I took advantage of opportunities. I had to overcome many difficulties because it's always more difficult for a woman to achieve things naturally. I took part in all the fights for women's rights, but there's a lot of prejudice towards women who are labelled as feminists". Jacqueline is married and has two grown-up children, but says: "I have been very lucky, my husband is also militant and supports feminism. We have fought together and the children received a culture which they wouldn't have had, if we had been stuck in an office".

6 - Simone, is responsible for research in health in a direction of the French Ministry of Work, Health and Social Affairs. She previously worked in the commissionership for the health plan, then for some years was part of the Minister of Health's Cabinet. She has grown-up children.

c) The Swedish
1 - Birgitta, economist by training, presently holds a top position in the County Councils Federation which is the central political organization of the Country Councils; her board of directors is made up of elected politicians. She is also chair of a large national organization involved in road and traffic administration, and about this she says: "I was nominated because this time there was a real desire to

have a woman, before there had only been men and a change was necessary". She has had a wide experience in other high level jobs in the Civil Service: for 15 years she worked in the Ministry of Finance as economist, then she was in Parliament, then with the Ministry of Transport and Communications, then head of traffic administration in her city and finally research director in a research institute on transport and communication. She comes from a very poor family, but her parents wanted their children to study and they made a lot of sacrifices to achieve this.

2 - Ingela, educated as an economist, she now holds a top political position at the Ministry of Health and Social Affairs. Previously she worked for the Ministry of Finance. She is young, not even 40 years old. Her parents are small farmers and there was no tradition in the family to study or go to university, but she and her brother and sister all went to university and have now very good jobs. She says it is very important for her to work with humanitarian objectives and she is also interested in international relations. The only obstacle to her career is the fact that she is so young and that many high level positions are taken by men in their 60's who all know each other and form a tight net.

3 - Yvonne is a County Commissioner and is responsible for the health services. She is also deputy-mayor of her city, member of the board of directors of the Housing Company and a member of the Swedish Institution for Development of Health Care, an institution which has the task of programming medical-health assistance. She did not go to university, but to high school and training courses. She is divorced and has a grown-up daughter, but feels that the family was not an obstacle to her career; there were some problems when her daughter was small and her husband was interested, like she was, in politics, but they used to take the child to their meetings and "luckily she loved to read". It was difficult though when she worked full-time and also had to look after the house in her spare time.

4 - Eva holds a top position in a nurses, laboratory technicians and obstetricians' union. She is a professional nurse with a university education and specialized in intensive care. She works in a large hospital complex in the intensive care unit. She is also involved in international co-operation in a solidarity association for Palestine. An important factor in her education was that as a child she was taught that all human beings are equal and should have equal opportunities. Besides, she was also educated to believe that you can do whatever you want if you are really determined and this gave her a lot of self-confidence. "I'm also very stubborn, she says, and I want to do lots of things. For me a position in itself has never been important, but I wanted to change things". She has no children, lives with a companion, who is also very busy, so she feels that if she had a child it would be a problem.

5 - Lena holds a top position at the National Board for Health and Welfare, an advisory body of the Ministry made up of a staff of experts who control and follow the development of the medical sector. Lena was trained as a cardiologist and previously was head of a research centre in a large university hospital. She was very successful both as a physician and in the research sector. Married, with three children, she says that it is very difficult to combine both family and work, also because in Sweden it's not easy to find paid help. Her husband "helps".

o o o

These brief profiles of 16 women holding important positions in the health service of their countries, show that these women are strong, extremely determined, and have committed themselves in their personal training far beyond their formal education including, in rare cases (Jacqueline and Yvonne) those who did not go to university. They are women who have had a rich professional career in different fields and who, apart from their work, have also taken on other social and associative responsibilities.

Nearly all have a family and children, often more than one. The fact of having family and children isn't seen as a restriction to their career in the case of the Swedish women who were able to take advantage of reasonably efficient child services and perhaps even "help" from their husbands (in spite of the fact that in this country, as some of them affirmed, it isn't culturally accepted to use paid home help). They feel, instead, that they are helped by a strong culture of equal opportunities and stimulated by their families to go ahead, even if the family is poor or from a lower social class.

This situation is quite different for the Italian and French women: the little understanding from husbands about women's professional career, the excessive work burden which includes "the double presence" and lack of collaboration in looking after children was the reason for divorce for at least three French and two Italian women and for the others involved great sacrifice in their career and personal stress, even if they found in their own will-power, the strength to continue with their career together with looking after a family and children.

4.3 Access to top positions and process of professional selection

Two French interviews revealed the contradictions existing in France between the constitutional principles of equality and the real situation: "There is still a lot of discrimination in this country - observes Jacqueline - none of the constitutional principles are applied. We currently face a contradictory situation: it is taken for granted that women have a right to equality, but in fact women have little access to positions of power. I think that power is an extremely perverse factor; many men hold onto their positions and are opposed to working under a woman". Also Thèrese talks of paradox and adds that even in the public sector which is "less sexist than the private one" there are few women in positions of power even when women are better than men because "to get there they have to be better". On the other hand, as Simone observes, in the French health sector, decision-making power at a government and even parliamentary level is very weak. Jacqueline, believes that health insurance is a male environment and that the presence of women in high positions is inversely proportioned to that represented at an occupational level: only in 1986 was the first woman elected on the board of directors of the federation she belongs to.

In spite of a greater presence, compared to other countries, of women in decision-making, two Swedish women respondents stress that, even in their country, the top positions occupied by women do not correspond to their effective occupational presence in the sector (Birgitta). Eva observes that although 50% of politicians in Parliament and in the County Councils are women, in hospitals 70% of hospital directors are men, as are most of the physicians.

If inequality persists in access to decisional power we must take a look at the reasons for this. In the first place, the interviewed women from all three countries underlined, though in different ways, the different prestige that medical professions still have if prevalently carried out by men or women. Even within the same profession, on the one hand a differing hierarchy of power is noted among the various specializations, on the other the process of selection is still conditioned by prejudices which in fact put women at a disadvantage.

Regarding this, one Italian respondent (Paola) remembers that half the students enrolled in medicine are women and that 40% among those who graduate, but then selection occurs: "In a career such as researcher or university professor there really is an obstacle, a prejudice. The class of physicians doesn't want women among them, selection is made by the university professors who are all men and favour their own sex: they choose who to give tasks and patients to. There are hardly any women surgeons because the chief surgeon chooses who will operate in his place and always chooses men; in paediatrics and other branches where the same patient can be seen by more than one physician women can gain experience, but in surgery women are excluded. Another reason why they are excluded is that a woman is less inclined to stoop to compromises than men, she won't close an eye to mistakes. Perhaps because we women have to work so hard to obtain a position and to conquer it by demonstrating that we are good, that we are then no longer willing to accept these things".

Another Italian, Elsa, reminds us that in Italy the professional independence of psychologists still hasn't been recognised, so that they have no right to management and find themselves in operative units directed by medical figures.

Simone observes that in France there is a very close knit hierarchy even in the kind of training you receive: the top positions in public management are occupied by people who come from ENA (Ecôle National d'Amministration), while the National School of Public Health mainly trains managing directors of hospitals and does not have great prestige.

Another French respondent, Thèrese, also refers to the diverse presence of women in the various medical professions. Nursing, she says, has prevalently been a female occupation and very underestimated; it is therefore right to vindicate respect for the profession. Where the medical profession is concerned, there are many women in fields such as anatomy, pathology, ophthalmology where work organization offers greater freedom; many are specialized in geriatrics or else in fields which don't have great prestige. "In France it has been found that when a respected and well-paid profession is trivialized, then the number of women who practice it increases; the medical profession was considered nearly sacred when there were few women in it, while now their number has increased and the physician's status has lowered. I think that the fact there are so few women surgeons is also due to a cultural factor which sees the woman as a protagonist in curing, but without using a knife. Women have always chosen to treat with herbs, will-power, potions...It's not a technical question linked to ability, it's cultural".

Regarding the loss of prestige of professions which become womanized, Danielle observes: "Often you hear it said that a profession loses prestige when it has as many women as men. The only way to overcome this obstacle is to have as many women as men everywhere". Catherine, stresses the existence of macho behaviour on the part of her male colleagues who, she says, "in the first place consider you a woman and then a colleague. It is rare to be trusted by your colleagues, you have to conquer both your own space and trust very slowly".

o o o

The subject of the diverse presence of women in various health professions is also taken up by the Swedish respondents. Ingela believes that also in Sweden there are differences: women make up more than half of the students in medicine, but only a fifth are professors; besides, even here stereotypes still exist and there are more female nurses than male, and more female general practitioners and more male surgeons. Lena adds that female medical students are treated differently by the professors than male ones and that certain specializations, such as cardiology, are considered to be male territory: "I believe, she adds, that in the Western world only about 7% of cardiologists are women, in Sweden the percentage has grown a little in the last few years, but it's still within 12-15%". To obviate these problems, the largest hospital centre in Stockholm has set up a "mentorship" programme for each new medical student to help him/her publish and attain university or other good working positions.

Birgitta believes that women don't reach top positions because they work in unqualified professions. In Sweden, she says, both males and females have the same possibilities of studying even if they come from a poor family, it is natural then that girls have an education and work and that housework is divided between boys and girls.

Eva, instead, puts more emphasis on the scarce appreciation of women's professions and knowledge rather than on women's educational choices: "In the medical sector there is a very strong tradition where only physicians have real knowledge and we nurses have had to fight so that what we knew could emerge and that those in decision-making roles in health would also listen to us as holders of a different kind of knowledge than physicians. In the medical sector there is medicine and there's the science of care, if more attention was given to caring there would be more women in decision-making. This, however, would be threatening to physicians, and the politicians don't want to interfere with the professions. Health is still a very hierarchical sector, nurses have a lot of responsibility in practical work, but very little formal power. I believe that work in health assistance is organized in such a way so as not to give nurses the possibility of using all their knowledge; they have been greatly undervalued and this has involved a waste of knowledge and money".

4.4 Involvement in the family and self-esteem

Elsa faces the subject of impact of the "double presence" (in work and in the family) on women from the point of view of her professional experience, that is of mental unease. It therefore seems right to start with her testimony. "The cause of difficulties that emerge in daily life is the same for different contexts: it is always the woman who has a burden of responsibilities which prevents her from following a career. Man is able to recuperate his energies in the family, the woman doesn't have this possibility and goes to work tired. Besides she is also limited by the absence for maternity leaves and by difficulties in going to training and up-dating courses. The very reason of not recognizing her double work and the legitimacy of being tired, leads the woman to consider her tiredness as a mental problem, as subjective inadequacy and not as a consequence of life conditions". Following this analysis, Elsa goes on to say that it is important to recognize that women's work burden is excessive and ask them to delegate to others, both in the family and at work. "Women don't have the strategy of pulling out of situations, so that they finish up by doing everything, get angry, are not thanked for what they do, get tired and then the symptom arrives and it's tragedy".

Also Paola believes that women give up taking on more responsibilities because they cannot reconcile the enormous work burden of management with family requirements. "The relationship with the husband is compared daily with interest for work; I have seen many female colleagues refuse tasks because their role as wife and mother couldn't be substituted. Instead, I believe that it's different when one has children, because especially when the child is small you can take him/her with you".

Anna stresses that, besides family responsibilities, other factors play an important part, such as: the fact of having to struggle hard in order to have a career and the widespread cultural attitude where women are supposed to be more family than work oriented. Where this point is concerned, she thinks that it is important to send different messages to women regarding work which can lead to a progressive growth of women".

Grazia points out the absence of services for small children and underlines the fact that in a city full of babies like hers, there are only three public crèches for a total of 120 babies. Moreover, opening and closing times of kindergartens and primary schools do not coincide with working hours and no-one has ever thought about resolving this problem.

o o o

Compared to most Italian regions, the services for small children in France are organized much better, but even here the dominating culture puts the burden of housework and looking after children on the woman. It's not by chance, then, that all the French respondents underline that looking after a family greatly restricts women's professional career.

Michéle, who is employed in numerous different professional and community activities, affirms that a woman's life changes completely when she has children and that the greatest obstacle for women is precisely lack of time. "The time we spend in a community organization we take from our family; we have to teach the father to baby-sit when the mother has a meeting in the evening. Another obstacle is the way men see women, their desire for power and their suspicion of how women manage politics: expertise being equal, women are always required to be better. Women have realized they have a role to play and day after day they have to struggle to impose themselves, believe in themselves and win trust from others. I don't believe much in quotas, the motivation comes from us; it's in a woman's character to say "I'll do this and then I'll see what the results are" and then "I managed it, now we can go on" and I see that we manage to gain a little bit of ground at a time like the sea on a beach".

Simone thinks that the obstacles are mainly subjective: women's poor self-esteem, their tendency to draw back, to ask themselves if it's "really worth the trouble", but she then admits that many women are really on their own when coping with the many concrete problems of educating their children, with time-tables.

Also Thèrese agrees that what prevents women from occupying positions of management is above all a subjective psychological condition: a more or less conscious conditioning which forces women to feel that looking after children and the house is a priority. It is incredible, she says, that when a man is left on his own with his children everyone considers him to be terribly unlucky, while when a woman is left on her own then she just has to get on with it. The danger, she warns, is the diffusion of part-time "which puts the woman in a situation of great economic submission and loss of power in an apparently comfortable way, while in the meantime, the "lords and masters" are involved in "serious matters". Thèrese believes that the path towards equality is very long, and that 2-3 generations are still necessary. A lot depends on the mothers, who still today don't push their daughters to positions of power. The aim must be equality, but there has to be equality right from the start: "If there aren't many women at the starting point, then there can't be many in higher positions. I don't believe in special measures which will allow women to have access, but in indirect measures such as, for example, giving nurses the management of nursing services".

Jacqueline also mentions women's underestimation of their own abilities, but above all she stresses that many men give no consideration to the responsibility of running a household and bringing up children. "If you consider - she says - that in our country there has been an increase of single parent families from 200,000 to 1,200,000 it is obvious that this poses some problems: women have to make a considerable effort to train themselves, be available and open-minded when left alone with children, but if one really wants to promote women to the same level of responsibility as men, then they must be given the means to do this, such as, for example, training in the work place".

According to Catherine, one of the major obstacles to women's career is the number of working hours required in the position of director or manager. "In France, - she says - a manager has to be willing to work 50 hours a week, until about seven in the evening, otherwise you are not considered to be serious. This is a huge obstacle for women with family responsibilities. Another obstacle is the public examinations which impose geographical mobility over the whole country; this does not always fit with family programmes and so one is forced to make difficult decisions".

○ ○ ○

It is certainly a mistake to say that the problems of women's double burden of both work and family do not exist in Sweden. However quite a different situation emerges from the interviews, compared to France and Italy. Even though the problem of lack of time for women also exists in Sweden, all our respondents underlined the important role which the culture of equality has played in that country and of the widespread services for small children.

"We believe - says Birgitta - that children need to be with other children. Here in Sweden one has the right to the "Day-Care Service" for babies; in any case 85% of married women with children work. It is normal for women to work outside the home, even if many work part-time". Birgitta also stresses that in Sweden every institution has to have by law an Equality Policy for men and women, also because it has been found that women have professionalities which need to be valued and that having women in top positions adds quality. For example, in the last few years mainly women have been nominated as hospital directors in Stockholm.

Still on the subject of infant service efficiency Ingela reminds us that Sweden, second only to Ireland, is the country where most children are born, and adds: "If it's true that women with careers have difficulty in combining maternity and work, then it is also true that young men have the same problem if they want to be good fathers".

Also according to Yvonne, child care in Sweden is not a problem because it is well organized, but she believes that lack of time is effectively a problem for women with a similar position to hers. She does remember, though, that sometimes rules do not correspond to women's requirements because they have been written by men and she gives the example of her City Council regulation which does not foresee temporary replacement of a council member for maternity reasons, therefore when this situation actually arose the regulation had to be altered to allow another women to substitute the one on maternity leave.

According to Eva, compared to other European countries, Swedish men participate much more in family work, even if the reponsibility is always the women's and the man "helps". "Studies have been carried out, she says, which show that when a man comes back home his level of stress falls, while when a woman comes back home her level of stress increases because she just goes on doing more work". Besides, according to this respondent, communities are starting to cut funds for the "Day Care Centres" and because of this many women work part-time: for example, in Sweden 53% of female nurses (compared to 19% male nurses) work part-time. Eva says though, that there's another reason which prevents women from taking on reponsibilities: lack of self-esteem which, for example, leads women to always underestimate their work when talking about it, while a man will describe it - even when it's the same work - as being much more complex. For this reason her union tries to do a lot of work on self-esteem and make women more aware of how important their role is and to be able to adequately describe their work. The union has also set up special negotiation courses for women to help them take on greater power.

Lena, instead, says that lack of self-esteem and motivation is not really a serious problem in Sweden as it is in other countries, at least for the new generation of women. The political work carried out up to now, she goes on to say, "has lead to a situation where it is considered quite normal that women should have their opportunities and decisional bodies with few women are looked on with suspicion". More than one Swedish respondent, mentioned that an important factor which helped them to increase their self-esteem, was the presence of someone in the family who encouraged them to be strong and independent.

4.5 The innovative contribution of women in health policies

The conclusions of the previous chapter underlined the importance of a balanced participation of women in health decision-making, not only for democratic reasons, but also because they brought with them new ideas, different kinds of priorities, different ways of dealing with problems and with the decisional processes. It was found that women in all European countries agreed on this. This has become even more evident for the in-depth interviews in this chapter: as we will see, even if women stress or underline different aspects, there is a great homogeneity of views among Italian, French and Swedish women.

According to Elsa women can bring about changes: as they have more contact with practical, everyday problems, they have acquired power and it is right that they should be able to "run the show". If, when choosing managers, you aim on productivity, then women's competence must emerge together with the "pluricapacity of looking at a whole" which women have due to their daily work burden. "A woman can do two, three things at once: do and think. Women's strength is not dividing material work from intellectual work". As an example of the different methods of women's intervention, Elsa talks about the method used by her team: first of all to listen to the patient, understand the primary causes of discomfort, early prevention and identification of risk factors, avoiding, where possible, use of drugs. She also adds: "Few male psychologists and physicians use our methods because they have the prejudice that behind a pathology there is always some organic problem which has to be treated using drugs".

Even Anna stresses the importance of women's presence at a decision-making level because of their innovative contribution and their capacity to listen. Then she dwells on the different way women organize services: "men tend not to have a community kind of organization, a woman who becomes director can introduce a new model: she can concentrate on the part which has been more neglected, on psychotherapy, on the gathering of data, on rehabilitation, (use of drugs is male). It is important to develop a different orientation in the organization of services; a woman manager can make it possible for caring to become the dominant modality in the service and that it be valued. Work organization in hospitals can be changed: users and operators can be listened to. Every morning we have a brief meeting. I work in this service, which isn't easy as it's mainly male, without imposing, but giving my example, just working, doing my job. Since I became director the men who work for me have changed their attitude".

Paola also believes that women can make hospital organization more efficient and more welcoming and that women would bring different cultures and priorities. A paradox emerges from her interview: "The commissions on bioethics (which must exist in every medical structure) are composed of men; therefore a commission which must decide on insemination, abortion etc. is totally male!"

On the different kind of leadership Grazia reports: "Men say "it's an order from the management", instead I would prefer it if everybody could collaborate in making decisions and carrying them out because then they would be convinced that that was the best solution". Grazia also feels that even in service organization, in assigning shifts, it is important to pay attention to a woman's requirements, to the fact that she has children and do what is possible to allow her to carry on her work. "If this woman has children and I with my management orders upset her activities with her children, then in five years time I'll find these children in family planning clinics, in a SERT (service for drug addicts, HIV testing). Understanding this means preventing from a distance".

According to the respondent, moreover, women face some problems from a different angle especially when referring to pregnancy and chidbirth, because women know what happens in these moments. Even where breast cancer is concerned a woman physician has greater participation with the patient, while for a man a breast is just another organ. Regarding childbirth, one of the problems is that women are not made welcome and there is always so much hurry: "as the delivery room can't be blocked for hours, a woman after six hours of labour is sent off for a caesarian section, while if she had been allowed more time she could have delivered normally. Italian data confirm an excess of unnecessary caesarian sections due to hospital organization and this doesn't happen in other countries". For these reasons the respondent is involved in training courses for male and female operators, to teach them how to welcome pregnant women. As for the priorities on medical policies, Grazia underlines the importance of babies, of the newly born: it is at this point that prevention of disabilities and marginalization begins. If due attention is not given to frail and socially deprived babies, they will become marginalized and we will later find them in hospitals, in the SERT, in crime and the girls in family planning clinics to abort while still terribly young. "We know the path these children follow, we could take charge of them, follow them and help them to avoid that path".

o o o

The reflections of the French respondents are very similar. Michéle and Jacqueline, for example, underline women's diverse sensitivity and their greater stress on prevention. For Michéle, women have a more practical outlook, they are more capable of listening, they have a greater tendency towards prevention; besides, they are also more determined and when they have an objective they go ahead with it. According to Jacqueline, women's different approach to problems, their sensitivity regarding health problems, prevention, marginalization, is a richness which must not be wasted.

Simone observes that the presence of women in high decision-making levels helps to favour the presence of other women in the same position, as the strong prejudices towards them disappear with experience. She also mentions that women in management have a completely new attitude towards efficient leadership and are also able to rule men. Although Simone believes that basically priorities are not different between men and women regarding medical-health policies, she does say that men stress the importance of introducing the latest medical technologies more often than women, while the latter underline the need to face everyday life regarding loss of health, and therefore the importance of prevention, assistance to the disabled and the elderly, of childhood diseases.

In affirming that women's experience in medical-health care can improve hospital services, Catherine observes that treatment has become very technical and dehumanized: "Female nurses and operators should bring humanity to medical environments, but often they don't do so because they would have to fight to impose this on the all-powerful physician". She adds that public health and prevention are strongly felt by women, who are able to evaluate long-term results, while men are more inclined to achieve immediate results. In fact, Catherine points out that France has still not been able to set up a series of efficient services for family planning, pregnancy and abortion.

Danielle dwells on the different style of leadership that women have: "Women - she says - are more considerate about the people they work with. In contacts between woman and woman, problems regarding the family are understood much better, and therefore the distribution of work tasks is more attentive. While men tend just to give orders, a woman takes the personal life of her colleagues into account and manages to create an environment of greater respect". Where drugs are concerned, Danielle observes that women take more psychotropic substances, because when a woman doesn't feel well she is immediately prescribed drugs, tranquilizers and often treated as hysterical.

Women's authority, according to Thèrese, is usually less rigid than men's and more inclined to listening, and relating to others: "Women tend to look more for results than how these results can be of personal benefit. Perhaps women have a more global vision of medical problems, are more worried about how the public health sector works and about accompanying measures, because they have always accompanied someone from birth to death. Birth and death have been confiscated from women by the male medicalization of these stages of life". Thèrese underlines how some medical fields which particularly concern women have not been adequately developed: this is the case of osteoporosis, menopause, and of old age of women who live longer, but their health is not sufficiently studied from the point of view of ageing well.

o o o

Regarding the subjects dealt with in the paragraph the replies of the Swedish respondents were generally similar to those of their French and Italian colleagues: even they underlined that women bring new methods of working and managing in the health sector and that their priorities are prevention. Some differences can be found in their stress on the importance of mixed groups so as to have a contribution of various experiences and in an awareness that even Swedish men have learnt to appreciate the way women work.

Birgitta summarizes the thoughts of the Swedish respondents when she says: "Most people in management positions and most men, have realized that women have qualities which must be valued and that if there aren't any women in top health positions this results in a loss of quality. It is good to have mixed groups because different ways of working and thinking are combined and this is very important. The fact of having women in top positions in the health sector adds quality to the organization. Women have a way of working which must be promoted, they work in a network, in groups, they try and reach agreements, are more democratic, while men have a more hierarchical method. In the past women in top positions used to copy the male style of leadership, because it was more difficult for women to reach the top and so they had to fight men with their same weapons, they really had to be tough; but when there are many women, as in the health sector, then we find quite normal women in top positions who have a more feminine approach to work and leadership." Birgitta also mentions research showing how men and women who have had heart attacks have been treated in different ways and she observes that medical and pharmacological research has for a long time concentrated more on men than on women.

This last point is also dealt with by Ingela who observes that: "Drugs have a different influence on men than on women because the chemistry of our bodies is different, but most therapies are elaborated on men. When drugs are tested, these tests are nearly always done on men, but as women's bodies are different, nobody really knows what effects these drugs will have on them".

Yvonne reveals that in the present way work is organized women in top positions often feel alone because they work in a different way, they need to talk to each other, to compare what they are doing and she adds: "We women don't think that we lose prestige only because we want to come to agreements, what's important for us is the result. Women express themselves differently from men, they speak a different language; sometimes I realize that I've said one thing, and that it has been interpreted as something completely different from what I meant. When men talk together I think they tend to read between the lines, while women are much more direct and men try to read between our lines, while there really isn't any hidden meaning in what we say". Yvonne, like the others, believes that women have different priorities in medical policies and that certain areas of medical assistance have been developed thanks to the presence of women in top health positions: for example in caring for the elderly, in treating the final years of life, pain, chronic diseases, in the best way possible. "These things - she says - are much more on the agenda if there are women in decision-making positions. In medicine, instead, there is a status hierarchy: brain surgery has the highest level of prestige, but treating chronic diseases has little prestige and when there are more women in decision-making, these areas of low prestige are dealt with much more".

Lena expresses the same concepts of the other respondents quoting research data which she has both from her present role and from her previous experience as research director in a university hospital. Research carried out on trainee physicians showed that, compared to men, women are more "popular" among patients because they dedicate more time and show greater understanding and patients think that it is easier to talk to women. Also: "all research demonstrates that women are more interested in the social and psychological aspects of a disease, while men concentrate more on general medical measures, on doing things, on intervening". Where drugs are concerned, Lena believes that there are no doubts that they have different effects on men and women, because the metabolism is different, the number of side-effects vary between men and women. Women take more medicines and are prescribed more sedatives and tranquillisers. All these things are common knowledge thanks to recent research which has taken into account the two genders.

Also Eva takes up the subject on the different effects that drugs have on the two sexes. She also believes that: "the reason why open heart surgery has such high prestige and that research in this field is more advanced than in others, is because more men have heart problems and more of them have been involved in decision-making positions. For this reason there has been a greater inclination to resolve men's health problems rather than women's; if men had to take the pill, for example, perhaps research in this field would have been carried out better". Like the others, this respondent confirms that women are not tied to the old schemes when resolving problems, but look for new ways and in management try to reach agreements.

o o o

It is not an easy task to summarize schematically the quantity of information gathered from the life experiences and knowledge of our respondents. Each one adds elements of personal truth to the overall picture and to that of her country. All describe the diverse starting points for women which make the climb towards decision-making positions more arduous: the lower prestige of the more womanized professions, the difficulties of being accepted in decision-making, of organization of work, the lack of time. However, where these subjects are concerned, the situation of the Swedish women seems much better than of the French and Italians. And this depends on better organization of services for small children, but above all on a deeper cultural change - even if still not completed - which has brought about greater equality between men and women. A cultural change which in Italy and France has still a long way to go.

The last part of the analysis has confirmed that all respondents hold a very similar view towards the importance of their role in public health: the deep awareness of bringing new ways of working and being leaders and of having different priorities in medical policies then men. Women look for results in time, rather than in the immediate present, they also look at specific female problems. If there is a difference among the respondents of the three countries, it is that in Sweden men have begun to appreciate the contribution of women. Also, in this country, medical and pharmacological studies have finally begun to take into consideration gender differences. This first important step is merit of the presence of women in decision-making processes in health.

Chapter 5

CONCLUSION AND PROPOSALS

If we were to make a synthesis of the main themes covered in our research, we would say that, first of all, it has analysed the unequal representation of men and women in health decision-making, then the factors affecting the female representation and finally the innovative contributions of women in health policies. Let us now, synthetically go through the main results of the research by inserting them in a more general view, with the help of relevant literature. We will conclude, then, with some suggestions drawn from the material collected and from the experiences referred to in literature.

5.1 Gender disparity in career opportunities

Our research has shown in the first place that, in spite of the large representation of women in all health professions, as far as equal access to decision-making is concerned there is still a long way to go in most European countries. The data collected during our research in the 15 countries of the European Union have shown that, in spite of a considerable representation of women in the political institutions of many EU Member States, the share of women in top positions is quite low in hospitals, in sickness funds, in consultation and bargaining bodies, in medical associations and unions. However, we found considerable differences among the three "major European regions" (North, Centre and South of Europe). As a matter of fact, according to our data, the participation of women at top decision-making levels is higher in the five North European countries, which are characterized by a "universal" model of health protection. It is lower, instead, in the six Central European countries - characterized by an "occupational" model - where the representation of women is particularly low in mutual associations and in sickness funds. In the four South European countries the participation of women to decisional positions shows, generally, the lowest rates, except for the public administrative bodies. In conclusion, the participation of women in decision-making is favoured by the public system of "universal" health protection.

Our sample survey (in which 220 women and 178 men participated) has shown that, compared to men, women are often disadvantaged in their career and in the access to power, because of: the selection criteria referred to for top positions, the un-equal allocation of tasks, the differential access to the informal networks and to "influential people", etc.

We found, however, some relevant differences: compare to Northern Europe, for instance, prejudices and discriminatory practices against women are more frequent in Centre and South of Europe. Moreover, in Central and Southern European countries, the double work load women are involved in - in professional work and in family caring - is a relevant obstacle for their access to decisional roles which imply a considerable involvement in terms of time. Often

41

these women are compelled to make difficult choices between family and their career or to cut down their aspirations. The relevant number of Central and Southern European women who are "single", divorced and without children is an indicator of the choices they are faced with; it seems almost that, in these countries, the fact of not having a family is a factor favouring the career of women.

The qualitative interviews of the Italian and French women in top positions confirm these results of the survey in a very lively manner. These interviews have also clearly shown that although the problem of lack of time exists for Swedish women as well, in Sweden family responsibilities do not inhibit the access of women to decision-making positions as frequently as in the other two countries. This is due to: the large availability of child care services, to the involvement - even if only partial - of men in family responsibilities and, mainly, to the diffused culture of equal opportunities in this country. The combination in Sweden of a high female activity rate with a high natality rate can be considered as a proof of all this.

o o o

As far as the obstacles to the women's access to top decisional positions, the results of our research are coherent in many aspects with the results of a study made in USA on career opportunities of men and women in health administration (Walsh, 1995). In the first place, also this research shows that, compared to men, a definitely higher proportion of women are "single" and without children, which - according to the author - could indicate that some women may be sacrificing their personal life for their career, while others with families may give up their career. Moreover, also this research has shown the importance, for career purposes, of interactions with senior managers, of knowing influential individuals within the organization, of informal networks; all variables, these, to which women have lesser access. In particular, women were found to have less interaction opportunities with those executives who can be vital for career development (because they can make the individual more visible, assign important projects, provide information about career prospects and provide access to informal networks).

With regard to the fact that women have less opportunities of access to information, to informal networks and rules, which are particularly important in public administration, it has been underlined that: "We register a wide discrepancy between the formalism of prescriptions and the informality of actual rules. The organization of public administration is defined by rigid and universalistic norms. In reality the organization works in a different and extremely informal way. As the discrepancy is so wide it becomes very difficult to decode the real functioning of the organization". In this situation women may be at a disadvantage on account of "the fact that they are particularly unprepared to face this lobbying, this infomal work, based on resources which are not those formally foreseen by the organization" (Beccalli, 1993, pp.67-68).

o o o

The sample survey as well as the qualitative interviews, clearly raised the argument of the differential participation of women in the various health professions: a lower share of women in the medical professions and a very high participation of them in the non-medical health professions in all the European Union countries. On this matter the Italian, French and Swedish women interviewed for the qualitative study underlined some relevant problems regarding access to power positions. First of all they underlined that the "feminization" of professions implies their de-valuation and loss of prestige. Secondly, they underlined the lower prestige held by the non-medical professions; particularly that of nurses, technicians and midwives, but also of psychologists, who - at least in Italy - are under the authority of physicians. According to the women interviewed, this leads to both an excess of representation of physicians in health decision-making and, at the same time, an under-evaluation of professions which have a more direct knowledge of reality and more ability in communicating with the patients. Also, there is, within the medical professions, a precise hierarchy of prestige and power among the different specializations. The Swedish women interviewed, as well as the French and Italian ones, all underlined this point. They also underlined, that women doctors have less opportunities of access to some medical specializations (in primis, surgery) because of the selection made by the male professors in favour of their same sex .

Regarding women practising such a demanding profession as the medical one, the respondents have shown the difficulties that those who have a family have to undergo; sometimes these difficulties may involve surrendering more gratifying roles. On this subject there is a wide bibliography for the European countries. Heuwing (1992), for instance, writes that at present, all over the world, 40-50% of medical students are women, but the percentage of women among practising physicians varies between 35 and 70%, being particularly high in East European countries where the medical profession is considered among those with the lowest prestige. The author underlines, moreover, that the difficulties in reconciling the medical profession with family responsibilities are common to all the countries, as are the strategies adopted by women physicians to overcome them (medical specializations and jobs with minor prospects, part-time, interruption of professional activity for more or less long periods). These strategies, however, often imply a retrenchment of their professional ambitions. As a consequence, women physicians are concentrated in "sheltered" specializations, such as psychiatry, anaesthesia, paediatrics. Moreover, according to Heuwing, the medical careers are often the outcome of personal acquaintances and of sponsorship of the young physicians by the network of older physicians. In Germany as well as in most European countries - according to this scholar - there are many good women students in medicine, they perform well in their studies, but their problems start when they try to build up their career both because of discriminations and because the medical profession requires a great deal of time.

Another German author (Muller, 1994) adds that relevant handicaps are the reduced geographical mobility of women physicians and the fact that rarely their husbands take some responsibility in child care. An Austrian author (Glatz, 1995), notes that while the share of women general practitioners increased consistently between 1981 and 1994, during the same period the increase in the share of women among medical specialists has been negligible, because women are systematically discriminated against at the moment of allocation of specialization posts. The share of women head physicians in Austria is only 8%.

A study held in Northern European countries (Korremann, ed., 1994), finally, underlined that women physicians are more often "single", that they have a more global view of the problems of the patient, they believe that tasks in the workplaces are unequally distributed among men and women, and they have minor managerial responsibilities. This study, instead, did not find significant gender differences as far as attitute to career and qualification are concerned, and in some areas men were found to be just as oriented towards the patient, the family and co-operation, as women are. Therefore, according to the authors, this research shows that - in the Northern countries - a phase of transition is being passed, where both men and women are moving closer to each other in their behaviour, in their perception of the job, of their career, of their professional values; however women's perception is that they encounter a system that sets up barriers against them.

o o o

Another theme relevant for our discussion of the disadvantages facing women in their access to decision-making bodies refers to the type of people required for those roles. More precisely, it is worth understanding whether women are chosen because they have attitudes and characteristics similar to men's, or for their specificity and for the innovative contribution they can give. On this argument, the conclusions of a Dutch study on the representation of women in advisory bodies are interesting. As the authors write: "Representation of women implies, in our view, arguments concerned with equality, as well as arguments concerned with difference. In the context of advisory bodies the gendered nature of expertise must be examined as well... The representation of women was an issue, but mainly as an aspect of equality, as a search for women who are "the same", "women of quality". Expertise in women was never seen as necessary and sometimes actively rejected. We concluded that ... women are represented, but only when they have become the same as men. .... However, the search for "the same" women sometimes results in finding "different" ones" (Oldersma and Janzen-Marquard, 1994, pag. 23).

5.2 Continuity and change: the contribution of women

The subject we have just treated introduces the theme of the role of women in health. I would like to point out, first of all, that our sample survey, as well as the French, Italian and Swedish women interviewed for the qualitative study, have shown that women think that - in those bodies where health policy decisions are taken - gender is just as important as competence and that, their participation in these bodies is important not only for a principle of equity, but also - above all - for the different way women have of confronting health problems and because of their wide experience of caring problems. Indeed, the women of the North as well as those of the Centre and the South believe that they have different views from men in health policy matters, a different style of leadership and that women contribute in a new and valuable way to change because they have a more global view, they resort to a method of work based on confrontation, on group or équipe work, and because they are able to listen to patients, to colleagues and to those working under their leadership. The result is a more effective health care due to their more global knowledge of the health-care problems and their better way of communicating. In conclusion, this approach is a wealth which must not be lost, but should be diffused.

A group of women in leading health position in Naples is working on these themes and has produced several documents. The documents maintain that women have acquired a competence on caring activity in the family and in the profession; this competence is not inborn, but acquired and may, therefore, be acquired by everyone; and that caring activity, rather than a job should be considered as a method and as such can be applied to all types of work and can be acquired by everyone. (Comune di Napoli, Gruppo Salute, 1996).

With reference to the different leadership style of men and women the results of a research on men and women who have been mayors of the same American cities are quite interesting (Tolleson-Rinehart, 1991). This research also showed that women give more importance to participation, to collegiality, to team-work and to communication. Moreover, according to the author, the very presence of women changes the appearance of political leadership; this means that with their growing presence in seats of political power, we can expect women and men to understand power and leadership in new ways.

o o o

Besides the innovative method of work and style of leadership, our research also underlined that women have, on their agenda of health policies, different priorities from men. They seem to give more importance to prevention; health promotion; integration between social and health services; caring of the elderly and of chronic diseases; and the need for giving a better life to those who have lost their health. Our respondents, moreover, underlined that women pay more attention to problems related with the maternity-infant sector, and more generally to all areas concerning specific female problems: pregnancy, childbirth, caring of the new born child, prevention of breast and womb cancer, menopause, osteoporosis, taking care of the ageing process in women. In synthesis, men seem to be more inclined to prescribe drugs, to medicalization, to resort to advanced technologies, to intervene on serious pathologies - heart attacks, brain surgery, etc. - which have more prestige in the medical hierarchy; women, instead, seem to have a wider view, seeking long term results, giving relevance also to low prestige areas.

Related to all this is the argument that very often pharmacological research does not take into account gender differences in its experiments, while there is no doubt that many drugs have different effects on men and women, because of their different metabolism. The Swedish women interviewed mentioned this problem, underlining that very often drugs are tested only on men; they mentioned also some researches attesting differences in curing men and women. I don't believe that the fact that these researches are particularly developed in Sweden is a mere coincidence. On the contrary, I believe that, if today gender difference is taken into account in medico-pharmaceutical research, this is due, at least in part, to the increase in the participation of women in health decision-making. Among other things, the indicators of health efficiency previously recalled showed a greater efficiency of the Swedish health system, with reference to the maternity-infant sector. On this matter, Eduards (1995, and quoted bibliography) recalls that several surveys held in Sweden have shown a correlation between a wide representation of women at the political-administrative level and the development of social services, in particular those for children. Eduards, moreover, recalls that several studies of North European Parliaments have shown that, wherever female problems are taken in consideration, there are women bringing them up in the political agenda.

o o o

It is worthwhile to recall, at this point, a very important data which came out both from our sample survey and from our qualitative study. Women in health decision-making, with their innovative contribution in the method of work, in the leadership style and in health political choices, have also produced a change in the behaviour of men. This was underlined particularly by the Swedish respondents with decisional roles. Moreover, due to the very fact that there is a wider representation of women in Sweden, these respondents, compared to their Italian and French colleagues, underlined with greater emphasis the importance of both men and women participating in health decision-making, because plurality is wealth and allows a global view.

On these last subjects, an American scholar (Tolleson-Rinheart, 1991), recalls that in Scandinavian countries, where the largest concentration in the world of elected women is found, the political choices have changed as well. The author maintains that the very presence of women has brought to everyone's attention problems once considered only women's concerns and concludes: "Women in elective office have brought attention to, and made a place in the public agenda for, problems that have almost always been with us, but that have not been seen as proper questions for political deliberation in the past. Now, through the efforts of women, these "women's" issues are increasingly recognized as issues affecting the well-being of the entire public" (page 101).

In conclusion, a more balanced representation of women in health decision-making is important not only for a question of equity in representation, but also, and above all, because women bring new values, new ideas and a new style and method in decision-making. Moreover, in those systems and countries, where, for some time now, women have played an important role in health decision-making, also men's attitude is now beginning to change in their favour; this means that the latter have had a chance to appreciate the importance of women's innovative contribution in the field of health policy.

5.3 What to do: proposals and examples of sound practices

It is relevant, at this point, to ask ourselves what strategies should be adopted to ensure an equal representation of women in health decision-making. Many suggestions on this matter may be found in our interviews, in the relevant literature on single subjects and from the practices experienced in several European countries.

In the first place, primarily in those countries where an equal opportunity culture is not yet enrooted, cultural initiatives apt to circulate knowledge about the existing disparities and about the practices used to overcome them are very important. Fundamental are general cultural actions such as: sensibilization campaigns; actions aimed at overcoming the widespread cultural stereotypes, also in the media, on health professions; actions in schools aimed at educating young people to a culture of equal opportunities for all; actions aimed at favouring the access of women to emerging professions. The Swedish example has clearly shown the importance of a widespread cultural orientation on behalf of equal opportunities.

In the second place, of course, adequate social services are needed for children, the elderly, and the disabled. For this purpose, our research underlined the importance of the social services set up in some European countries. Sweden, for instance, has set up a widespread net of services for the elderly and for children (with pre-school activities for children of 18 months and over). Moreover, in this country the family policy includes 12 paid months for maternity leave; 450 days for parental leave for each child, under 8, one portion of which (90 days) must be divided between the mother and the father. (In 1989, 45% of fathers were using the parental benefit system, while in other countries - as in Italy, for instance - even if foreseen, the percentage of fathers taking advantage of parental leaves is irrelevant). Since 1983 the Swedish Government has implemented a number of projects, seminars, publications, group-works, training programmes for military conscripts, with the aim of stimulating fathers to take advantage of parental leaves. All this has favoured the Swedish high natality rate.

Similar initiatives could be very important to implement a deep cultural orientation in the countries still dominated by a traditional male culture. As I had occasion to underline elsewhere (Vinay, 1995), on these matters Public Institutions responsible for education, professional training and vocational guidance could do quite a bit. They could play an important role, moreover, in networking groups of women and health professionals using new methods of work in health, with the aim of implementing, through training and information, the use of these methods among colleagues. The City Council of Naples promoted a similar initiative by networking a group of women holding positions of responsibilities in local health institutions; requesting the local health administration to train health professionals taking into account the feminine specificity, to implement the women's model of work, to make the most of their abilities and to promote women's participation in decisional positions.

The practice of group work, of net-working is suggested also by the British National Health Service (NHS) not only as a means of obtaining better efficiency of the health system, but also as a means of exchanging information, developing career opportunities for women health professionals, strengthening women's self-esteem and increasing their collective strength.

o o o

Other actions could involve changing selection criteria and specifying clear targets to be reached in government appointments, in appointments for advisory and consultative bodies. For instance, in 1988 the Swedish government adopted a programme in three phases: 1) to make the shortage of women visible by means of a special inquiry and by means of annual statistical reports; 2) to establish concrete time-specific goals to increase the proportion of women on State boards and committees (30% in '92, 40% in '95), the final goal being equal male-female representation; 3) to pursue action that helps achieve these goals. The new procedures, among others, are going in this direction: every organization participating in State Commissions or bodies must provide two names for every position - a man and a woman - in this way the Government is able to appoint balanced bodies.

Similarly, the British National Health Service has promoted a wide action programme to favour the access of women in managerial positions setting concrete time-specific goals. This programme - called Opportunity 2,000 and launched in 1991 - followed a wide study on the innovative contribution of women in health management. During the first period of implementation of this programme (1991-1994) the rate of women managers has increased from 18% to 28% only two percentage points below the established goal. New specific numerical goals have been set for the second period of implementation of the programme (1995-1998), among, which, for instance, the increase in the rate of women managers to 35%. Moreover, many pamphlets have been published to inform women in the different health professions of career opportunities.

Also in Ireland the Second Commission on the Status of Women (1993) - having recognized that there is a significant under-representation of women in decision-making on Irish Health Institutions - asked the Ministry of Health to implement a programme which - among other things - sets specific numerical goals and to take into account gender balance in appointments for advisory bodies and for hospitals (at least 40%).

o o o

Political parties on their side should take their responsibilities. In Sweden, for instance, at least some of them have assumed the principle that every other name in the electoral list should be a woman's name; in this way an increasing number of women has been elected in Parliament and in regional and local administration. According to Eduards (1995), this type of self-regulation of the Swedish political parties may be due to the threat of a women's organization (Strodstrumporna) to build a women's party which according to the polls could have reached 40% of votes (both of women and men) in the 1994 elections. In any case, this self-regulation in preparing the elctoral lists could be an example for those countries which, in spite of their democratic tradition, still today have a very low representation of women in their Parliament and, as a consequence, also in health committees.

Also unions and medical associations should pursue the goal of a balanced representation of both sexes at top level. The Swedish union of non-medical personnel (nurses, laboratory technicians, midwives) has taken actions to encourage women to take leading positions, (special training programmes on negotiating and on self-esteem). For this purpose, we think it proper for the authorities in charge of selection of health managers to take into account also professionalities which are different from the medical ones (as psychologists, nurses etc.), because the knowledge these workers have, is a wealth which should not be wasted and which could contribute to better health organization.

As a matter of fact, the value and prestige granted to each health profession should not be considered as absolute and unchangeable. As has been written (Beccalli,1994), indeed the value attributed to the different professions is defined, by culture, by social relations, by power relations. It is not wrong, therefore, to redefine the actual hierarchy of values, also because the so-called "objectivity" on the basis of which it has been built, could probably have been vitiated by the unequal representation of men and women and by a power relationship which up to now has been in favour of men.

o o o

The problem of time is relevant for everyone, but, as we have seen, particularly for women; for this reason it is important to reorganize the time of work, finding forms of flexibility favourable to women, without penalizing their career opportunities. On this subject there are numerous suggestions with particular reference to physicians.

Research on North European women physicians, to which we have previously referred, in the conclusions recommends, among other things, more flexible working time structures, such as: staggered working hours, shared posts, part-time schemes, leave schemes and work-sharing. Similar suggestions have also been made by the Commission on the Status of Women (1993) for the Irish Health Institutions. Heuwing (1992), in the above mentioned article, also suggests introducing the opportunity to work part-time at all medical professional levels.

In Germany, in 1994, the annual Congress of the Association of Dependent Physicians (Marburger Bund, 1994), underlines that there are still numerous unsolved discriminations and structural problems impeding equal opportunities among physicians of the two sexes and that women, because of the difficulties of reconciling family responsibilities and profession, end up by choosing work posts incoherent with their expectations. For these reasons the Marburger Bund has approved a recomendation, asking a reduction of over-time work in hospitals, to comply with the requests of medical personnel to work part-time and to modify the actual norms in order to allow part-time work also in general practice.

Forms of flexibility of work-time are considered also by the British National Health Service in several publications of the project Opportunity 2,000. After underlining the risks for career development of the choice of part-time work by women physicians, it suggests that some forms of flexibilization of the time of work are apt to reduce these risks. This is true in particular for work-sharing, that is the possibility for two individuals to share the responsibilities of a full time post, sharing the time of work. This system (according to the NHS) allows to work fewer hours while retaining the status, benefits and career prospects of a full time post.

o o o

In the publications connected to Opportunity 2,000 reference is made also to another practice apt to promote career opportunities for women physicians: the introduction of "mentors" that is the practice of giving to senior physicians the responsibility to take interest in a more junior doctors' career development. An example of this practice was referred by one of our respondents: a mentoring programme which, in a large Swedish institution had positive results in increasing the number of women among medical university professors. Other similar experiences have given good results: the women who had taken part in these projects had acquired more self-confidence, a better understanding of their role and the capability to take greater responsibilities. Moreover, through this project, men had the chance to discover how different the language of women is. (Swedish National Institute of Occupational Health, 1994).

Coherently with the results of her research, Walsh (1995) also suggests resorting to mentors, who can provide a pragmatic framework that can guide the individual within both the health care organization and the profession and at the same time can facilitate interpersonal relationships which her research has shown to be so important for managerial career in health institutions. It is worthwhile to recall, in the end, as far as mentoring is concerned, that it is important for women to have other women as mentors in order to avoid reproducing, through male role models, leadership and work styles which normally are characteristic of men, thus reducing, from the beginning, the possibilities of change.

For this purpose I would like to mention that the Swedish women interviewed related the relatively high representation of women in decision-making in Sweden, noting that it has been a very long process, which is mostly due to the participation of women in politics who have created a support system for the working woman and good child care services. Moreover, they underlined the importance of the culture of equal opportunity which is now well enrooted in the country. However, according to some of the respondents, even if the conditions of women in Sweden are better than those in other European countries, this does not mean that all problems have been solved, because some invisible obstacles, "the glass ceilings", are still present also in this country, particularly in the academic world and in the private sector of economy.

o o o

The last argument I would like to mention has to do with the importance of statistical data collecting by sex, and with the importance of researches which have made it possible to know states of unequal power allocation, to understand the similarities or differences in the behaviour of the two sexes, in medical practices, and in the reaction to pharmacological products. We have mentioned numerous researches carried out in the different countries and particularly in Sweden. These researches have been mentioned also by our Swedish respondents, who asserted that the Swedish Authorities responsible for research and for pharmacological control have developed specific programmes apt to verify gender differences and to act accordingly. Without knowledge it is not possible to take adequate actions, research produces information, and knowledge is the first step towards change and towards a cultural reorientation of society.

I shall recall, on this matter, that several of our respondents, both regarding the sample survey and the qualitative study, greatly appreciated our research. This is, for instance, what an Italian respondent said:

> "This attention given to women is very interesting; it is one of the first times that there is this interest in a woman's way of thinking, in her professionality. This represents a gleam of hope in which we can see a new view of the system; we can see a wider perspective and we can see that, professionalities and competences being equal, putting the two roles together, we can obtain, perhaps, a clearer and more realistic view of problems".

A Swedish respondent said:

> "I think that your research is very interesting. I think that the very fact that you are doing such a research will contribute to having a larger number of women in decision-making; it will be very interesting to see the results".

From our side we "hand over" these appreciations to the Unit for Equal Opportunity of the European Commission who asked for this study. We recall that the contribution of the Union is very important to promote research, the circulation of information, of sound practices (which are objectives of the Fourth Action Programme) and the commitment undertaken with the Maastricht Treaty on Public Health matters (Title X, article 129) to implement actions, make recommendations and promote the co-operation among the Member States.

BIBLIOGRAPHY

Berthod-Wurmser M. (ed.), *La santé en Europe*, La Documentation Française, Paris. 1994.

Beccalli B., "Le azioni positive e l'amministrazione pubblica", in AA.VV., *Le azioni positive: un primo bilancio - Quaderni della Fondazione Malagugini,* F. Angeli, Milano, 1993.

Beccalli B., "Comparable Works", in *Pari e Dispari*, giugno 1994.

Eduards M., "Participation des femmes et changement politique: le cas de la Suède", in Ephesia, *La place des femmes. Les enjeux de l'identité et de l'égalité au regard des sciences sociales,* Paris, 1996.

European Network of Experts, *Women in Decision-Making* - Facts and figures on women in political and public decision-making in Europe, 2° ed., 1994.

European Parliament, *Il sistema sanitario negli Stati membri della Comunità europea. Analisi comparativa*, Direzione generale degli studi, W-4, Strasburgo, maggio 1993.

Federation of Swedish County Councils (Lena Eckerstrom), *Women Managers and Politicians in Swedish County Councils.* Stockholm, 1996.

Federation of Swedish County Councils, *Equality Policy*, Landstings Forbundet, Stockholm, 1996.

Ferrera M., *Modelli di solidarietà, Politica e riforme sociali nelle democrazie*, Il Mulino, Bologna, 1993.

Ferrera M., *The Southern welfare states in social Europe*, 1995, draft.

Flora P.-Heidenheimer A.J. (ed-s), *The development of Welfare States in Europe and America.* New Brunswick, Transactions, 1981.

Flora P. (ed*.), Growth to limits. The Western European Welfare States Since World War II.* volume 4 (appendix), de Gruyter, New York, 1987.

Gilley J. (ed.), *Women in General Practice*, General Medical Service Committee (BMA). London, 1994.

Glatz E. - Krajic K., *Berufschancen von Frauen im Gesundheitswesen*, (Gesundheit/ Krankheit). Statistical Yearbook, Wien, 1995.

Granaglia E., "Intervento pubblico e politica sanitaria", in P. Lange - M. Regini. *Stato e regolazione sociale. Nuove prospettive sul caso italiano*, Il Mulino, Bologna, 1987, p. 304.

Greek advisory committee on health, Ministry of Health, *Report on the Organisation and Management of Health Services in Greece*, Background material, Athens, april 1994.

Gruppo Salute - Assessorato alla Dignità - Comune di Napoli, "Materiali del sottogruppo sulla salute mentale", in *Atti del Convegno "Le donne nei luoghi decisionali"*, Roma, 16.2.1996.

Haut Comité de la Santé Publique, *La santé des Français*, La Découverte, Paris, 1995.

Heuwing M., "Arztinnen: Uberall und imme mehr", in *Deutsches Arzteblatt*, " August 1992.

Korreman G., *Laeger og koen spiller det en rolle?*, TemaNord, Nordisk Ministerrad. Kobenhavn. 1994.

INSEE, *Les femmes*, Service des droits des femmes, Paris, 1955.

Institute of Public Administration, *Administration Yearbook and Diary*, Dublin, 1995.

Jacobsson R. and Alfredsson K., *Equal Worth*, The Swedish Institute, Trelleborg, 1996.

Jones C., *Patterns of Social Policy. An introduction to comparative analysis* (chapt. 9: "Health Care"), Tavistock publ. London, 1985.

Marburger Bund, *"Klinik, Karriere, Kinder - Arztinnen Zwischen Anspruch und Wirklichkeit"*, Beschluss Nr. 1, Koln, 5.11.1994.

Muller S., "Familiengerchte Arbeitszeiten und Flexible Kinderbetreuung fur Artzinnen" in *Arzte Zeitung*, 12 November 1994.

NHS Women's Unit, *Making your Career in Medicine*, Department of Health, London, 1995.

NHS Women's Unit, *Managing beyond Gender. An Exploration of new management in the NHS*, Department of Health, London, 1994.

NHS Women's Unit, *Women in the NHS. Opportunity 2000*, Department of Health. London. 1996.

NHS Women's Unit, *Mentoring. A Guide*, Department of Health, London, 1996.

NHS Women's Unit, *Job Share. A Guide*, Department of Health, London, 1996.

OECD, *The reform of health care. A comparative analysis of seven OECD countries*, Paris, 1992.

OECD, *Les systèmes de santé des pays de l'OCDE. Faits et tendances*, 1960-1991. 2 voll., OECD, Paris, 1994.

Oldersma J., *The political construction of expertise*. Dep.t of women's Studies. Un. of Leiden, 1992.

Oldersma J. - Janzen-Marquard M., *Has Socrates risen?* Paper prepared for the conference: "Women and Public Policy: The Shifting Boundaries Between the Public and Private Domain" december 8-10, Leiden, 1994.

Statutory Office, *The Second Commission on the Status of Women Report to Government*, Dublin. 1993.

The Swedish National Institute of Occupational Health, *Women's Work and Health*, in Forskning and Praktik (English Edition), 1994.

Tolleson Rinehart S., "Do Women Leaders Make a Difference? Substance, Style and Perceptions", in *Gender and Policymaking. Studies of Women in Office*, Rutgers , University of New Jersey, 1991.

Vinay P., "Verso la parità nel lavoro e nella vita", in *Prisma*, 37, March, 1995.

Vinay P."La differenza di genere nell'approccio al lavoro e alla ricerca scientifica", in David P., *Donne all'Università*, Istituto Gramsci Marche, Tecnoprint, Ancona, 1992.

Vinay P. - Prospecta a.r.l. Ancona, *Women in Decision-Making in the Health Institutions of the European Union*, European Commission, V/5806/97, April 1997.

Walsh A., "Gender Differences in Factors Affecting Health Care Administration Career Development" in *Hospital and Health Services Administration*, 40:2, Summer 1995.

European Commission

Gender, power and change in health institutions of the European Union

Paola Vinay

Luxembourg: Office for Official Publications of the European Communities

1997 — 54 pp. — 21 x 29.7 cm

ISBN 92-828-1362-2

Price (excluding VAT) in Luxembourg: ECU 15